PHYSICIAN
ON A
MISSION

Dr. Veltmeyer's Rx to Save America

PHYSICIAN
ON A
MISSION

DR. VELTMEYER'S RX TO SAVE AMERICA

DR. JAMES VELTMEYER

LIBERTY HILL PRESS

Liberty Hill Press
2301 Lucien Way #415
Maitland, FL 32751
407.339.4217
www.libertyhillpublishing.com

Printed in the United States of America

Paperback ISBN-13: 978-1-6628-0876-0
Hard Cover ISBN-13: 978-1-6628-0877-7
Ebook ISBN-13: 978-1-6628-0878-4

TABLE OF CONTENTS

Dedication ix
Acknowledgments xi
Preface xiii
Introduction xv
Health Care: 1
Universal Catastrophic Coverage: Will It Work?. 3
"Right To Try" And Saving Lives 7
Medicare For All: Just Another Form Of Bureaucratic
Control 11
Employer Health Insurance: An Idea Whose Time
Has Passed 15
Reducing The High Cost Of Health Care 19
America's Coming Doctor Crisis: It's Already Here 23
Can Americans Trust The CDC? 27
Big Pharma: A Monster That Needs To Be Tamed 31
The Coming Medical Revolution. 36
Hospital Price Transparency: A Necessary First Step 40
Covid-19:. 45
A Viral Takedown Of Donald Trump. 47
Do We Permit A Virus To Destroy Our Economy? 51
Are We Being Misled Concerning Covid-19 Deaths? 55
Are State Lockdowns Legal?. 60
Unmasking The Dangers Of Face Masks 64

Entering The Post-Covid Era 68
The Verdict Is In: The Lockdowns Didn't Work 72
Quadramune For Preventing And Beating Covid-19 76
The Truth About Anthony Fauci 80
Covid: The Great Destroyer Of Liberty 84
Is The Covid-19 Vaccine The Answer? 88
Economy: **93**
Shattering The Myth Of "Free Trade" 95
The Hidden Hand Of Inflation 100
Rolling Back The Regulatory State 104
It's Time To Get Control Of Federal Spending 108
It's Time For Genuine Tax Reform 112
Government Action Can't Save The Economy 116
The Arrival Of "Hard" Socialism 120
Foreign Policy: **125**
Russia: The Enemy We Have Made 127
Toward A New Realism In Foreign Policy 132
Donald Trump And Endless Wars 136
The Taxpayer Rip-Off Called "Foreign Aid" 140
The China Syndrome 144
Immigration: **149**
Immigration Reform That Works 151
Immigration And The Nation-State 156
It's Time To Terminate The H1-B Visa Program 161
The Health Care Costs Of Open Borders 165
Democratic Party **171**
Democratic Party Elites Are The Modern Slave Masters 173
Has The Democratic Party Gone Crazy? 177
Democrats: The Party Of Infanticide 182
The Third Democrat Presidential Debate 186
It's Time To Recall Gavin Newsom 189
Democrats: The Party Of Racial Politics 193
Would JFK Recognize His Party? 198

President Trump: **203**
   Trump: Existential Threat To New World Order 205
   Impeachment: The Left's Fall Fantasy. 209
   Trump 2020: The Road To Re-Election. 213
   Trump And The Liberation Of The Republican Party . . . 218
   The Electoral College Must Save The Republic 223
   Theft Of An Election Or Theft Of A Nation?. 227
Republican Party: **231**
   GOP Establishment: Enemy Of The Trump Agenda 233
   The "Neo-Conservatives" And The GOP 238
   The New Political Realignment. 242
Federal Judiciary: **247**
   Dare We Defy Our Judicial Overlords?. 249
   A Polarized America And The Fourteenth Amendment. . 253
Culture:. **259**
   Mass Shootings: Sign Of Societal Collapse. 261
   The Cultural Marxist Attack On Western Society 265
   A Tale Of Two Americas 270
   Chaos In America: The Soros Blueprint 275
Education:. **281**
   Let The Free Market Solve The Crisis Of Higher
   Education 283
   Universities: Hotbeds Of Cultural Revolution. 288
Media: **293**
   It's Time To Break Up Big Media 295
Homelessness:. **299**
   Overcoming The Tragedy Of Homelessness 301
Federal Reserve System: **305**
   Is Trump Right To Go After The Fed?. 307
Deep State: **311**
   Is It Time To Abolish The CIA?. 313
Climate Change:. **317**
   Climate Change And Backdoor Socialism. 319

Social Security: **323**
   Quo Vadis, Social Security? 325
Law Enforcement: **329**
   The Hidden Agenda Behind "Defund The Police" 331
Public Employee Unions: **335**
   It's Time To Rein In The Public Employee Unions 337
Electoral Reform: **341**
   Mandating Election Integrity 343
The Biden "Presidency": **349**
   January 20, 2021: The Fall Of The Republic 351
   Resist Or Submit? 355
Dr. James Veltmeyer **359**

DEDICATION

To President Donald J. Trump,
The rightful winner of the 2020 presidential election
And, to my children, Olivia and Landon,
That they may continue to live in a free nation

ACKNOWLEDGMENTS

FIRST AND FOREMOST, I WOULD LIKE TO THANK MY longtime colleague and brilliant wordsmith, Andrew Russo, for all he has done to make this book a reality. I am grateful for his ideas, insight, wisdom and collaboration.

In addition, I would like to thank my wife, Laura, for her steadfast support and encouragement in this endeavor and her unsurpassed courage and optimism in the face of her ongoing health challenges.

I am also indebted to Mr. Benjamin Jones and Art World Gallery of El Cajon, CA, for the unique and striking front cover picture and design.

Finally, I thank my mother for all her sacrifices and for all she has done for me throughout the years, including her decision to send me to live in the greatest nation in the history of the world.

PREFACE

M ANY PEOPLE HAVE ASKED ME ABOUT THE ORIGIN of the photograph on the front cover. It's an 1891 painting by Luke Fildes that portrays a Victorian-era physician observing a child at a critical stage of illness. This picture has always reminded me of a deep personal experience as a child in Ecuador, when my younger brother was desperately sick with tetanus. We lived in a small two-bedroom apartment without electricity. All we had to light our small flat was candles. Fortunately, we lived near a hospital. A doctor carrying an aged medical bag came to our door and was led to the first bedroom, where my brother rested. I watched along with my siblings as he leaned over my brother, contemplating how to save him. And save him he did, thankfully. I have carried that image in my mind since that day. And, it reminds me of the Luke Fildes painting. I asked my illustrator, Benjamin Jones, to adapt the picture to show America as the bedridden child needing to be saved with the Father of our Country, George Washington, standing nearby. There is also the image of the child's mother — head in hand — if you look closely.

This picture embodies my mission to heal this great land at a time when it is suffering from what often seems to be an incurable malady, a sickness of cultural and moral disorder and decay that permeates and eats away at the very foundations of our constitutional republic, our "One Nation Under God."

It is my hope and prayer that the essays and commentaries in this book can provide the healing remedy (through the power of words and knowledge) that can restore the health of our nation, return it to its founding principles, and strengthen it against its numerous enemies both foreign and domestic.

INTRODUCTION

I'm Dr. James Veltmeyer. I came to America alone at the age of eleven when my mother decided that the only way I could have a better life would be to leave my nation of birth, Ecuador, and come to live with extended family in greatest nation on earth. The hunger, deprivation, and homelessness that I experienced in Ecuador only made me appreciate my new country even more.

Realizing the American Dream and climbing the ladder of opportunity in the U.S. allowed me to attain my life's ambition of helping others as a physician. Little did I know how much the cancer of government control, regimentation, and socialism that I saw growing up in the streets of South America had taken over our own health care system, once the finest in the world. I learned that not just as a doctor treating others, but I saw that cancer invade my own household (both metaphorically and in reality). Let me explain:

In 2015, my wife Laura was diagnosed with breast cancer. Her five-year long and counting battle with this dreaded disease and our personal experience with the worst aspects of government-run health care (i.e., Obamacare) sparked my desire to inform and educate the American public about the issues discussed in these commentaries and essays and to become involved in the political process, including as a Republican nominee for U.S. Congress in 2016. Laura's battle with cancer (which has subsequently metastasized to the lungs, bones, brain and other tissues) now requires experimental drug treatments and daily chemotherapy. This might not have happened had the axis of government and giant health insurers not come together under the Affordable Care Act to veto necessary early diagnostic testing at a stage when the cancer might have been stopped in its tracks. As a doctor, I was fortunate to have access to medical resources probably unavailable to many others – including leading oncologists. Yet, under the Obamacare regime, the expert advice of medical professionals is often overruled and approval denied for expensive, life-saving testing or treatments. This is what happened to my wife as she was denied – over and over again— for necessary tests and treatments despite our paying some of the highest premiums for the best policies on the market! It is a miracle that she is still alive today and we pray that her current treatments will be successful.

While the plurality of these essays do indeed discuss health care and the pandemic, many others address the other serious issues inextricably tied to what is happening in our country today, a nation torn by division, hostility, hatred and violence where our people seem to no longer share the fundamental values that gave birth to our free republic.

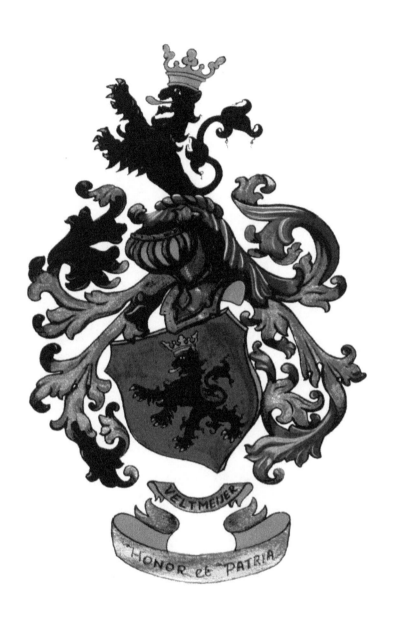

HEALTH CARE:

UNIVERSAL CATASTROPHIC COVERAGE: WILL IT WORK?

January 15, 2019

THE RECENT DECISION BY TEXAS FEDERAL JUDGE Reed O'Connor, striking down the so-called "Affordable Care Act" (aka Obamacare), offers Washington policymakers of both parties a unique opportunity to revisit the entire health care debate and craft a new plan that will actually improve people's lives while controlling costs. We should look back several decades for a possible solution.

In 1971, Harvard Professor Martin Feldstein, who later went on to be President Reagan's chief economic adviser, proposed a possible way out of America's seemingly intractable health care dilemma. It was called Universal Catastrophic Coverage (UCC) and its objective was to provide all people with health care coverage when they really need it, in life-threatening emergencies or major bankruptcy-inducing medical events, like cancer, heart disease, and newborns with genetic defects. UCC was not intended to cover the costs of routine or preventive care, like annual checkups, basic blood tests, sore throats, or runny noses.

3

No less than the great University of Chicago and Nobel Prize-winning free market economist Milton Friedman endorsed UCC in 2004 in an article he wrote for the Hoover Institution.

Under one version of Universal Catastrophic Coverage, all individuals not eligible for Medicare or Medicaid would receive a uniform, high-deductible catastrophic health insurance policy from a private company. The level of the deductible would be based on family income. The higher one's income, the higher the deductible. UCC would protect people from financial ruin in case of a devastating health care event, while allowing individuals to purchase "supplemental" insurance (such as Medicare recipients do) to pay for routine medical expenses. They could also rely on their health savings accounts or on a monthly membership in a direct primary care (DPC) provider practice. The estimated cost of such a universal catastrophic policy: about $2,000 a year or $160 per month. The vast majority of individuals would pay for this themselves, potentially using savings from the elimination of employer-paid coverage and higher wages. Those who cannot afford this amount would receive a voucher from the government to pay for it.

Membership in a DPC practice would permit individuals to contract with a direct primary care physician of their choice for a low monthly fee to access basic medical care, including 24/7 access to the doctor through unlimited office visits, e-mail and text, lab tests, x-rays, and even some medications. There would be no co-pays or deductibles. The monthly fees might vary, but are normally in the range of $50 to $100 per month per patient. Obviously, older patients who need to see their doctor more often would be charged at the higher end of that scale and younger people at the lower end. Children are even less, sometimes as low as $10 or $20 per month. Patients seeing their direct primary care provider on a regular basis (as there is no per office visit

charge but only the monthly fee) are less likely to be hospital-
ized, have surgeries or be admitted to the ER. Doctors are free to
spend additional time with their patients as they are not burdened
with answering to insurance companies or filling out reams of
paperwork.

While anyone can see that the direct primary care model
is highly affordable, does the same hold true of Universal
Catastrophic Coverage? The answer is yes, according to a study
by Kip Hagopian and Dana Goldman published in *National
Affairs*. Their analysis indicated that their version of UCC would
cost about half as much as Obamacare is expected to cost over
ten years ($950 billion versus $1.8 trillion under Obamacare).
Obamacare exploded the cost of health insurance by imposing
massive regulations and requirements on insurers to offer coverage most people did not want or need (i.e., single unmarried
men required to buy maternity or gynecological coverage, etc.).
UCC and direct primary care end that by creating a system where
catastrophic health insurance works hand-in-hand with a direct-
payer model for routine and preventive medical expenses without
breaking the bank. In some ways, it is similar to the much-praised
health care system in Switzerland. Unfortunately, the Affordable
Care Act virtually eliminated the option of catastrophic insurance
for anyone over thirty years of age, which is akin to eliminating
fire insurance for your home.

The price tag of UCC would be paid for by eliminating the
massive $250 billion tax subsidy for mostly large employers who
supply employer-paid insurance. UCC and direct-payer working
in tandem could largely supplant work-based insurance and allow
wages and salaries to increase instead, while freeing employees
from the chains of staying in jobs they dislike just to receive the
health benefits. Employers would also see the costly burden of
providing and administering health insurance lifted from their

shoulders. The entire system of employer-paid health insurance (tracing back to Bismarck's Germany in the 19th century) has served as a powerful disincentive for individuals to be personally responsible for their own medical needs – leading to overconsumption of high-priced services, such as the ER and hospitals for care that could be performed less expensively in a direct primary care physician's office, for example.

The beauty of Universal Catastrophic Coverage is that it returns insurance to its original purpose: protecting us in case something cataclysmic happens. The beauty of the direct primary care model is that it provides for all our other basic medical needs at a low, monthly fee, which can be accessed by both Medicare and Medicaid patients as well. The massive costs that physicians now bear for administrative, billing, coding and the rest will be drastically diminished as the role of health insurance companies will be carefully confined and corralled, no longer reaching out to interfere with medical decisions or line their own pockets.

Imagine the cost of your entire health care plan for $200 to $300 a month. It's time for health care *by* the people and *for* the people now!

"RIGHT TO TRY" AND SAVING LIVES

March 4, 2019

A LTHOUGH IT HAS DRAWN FAR LESS PUBLIC ATTEN-tion than the battle over illegal immigration, trade wars, North Korea or Supreme Court appointments, the Trump Administration is quietly initiating a revolution in health care. This administration's more decentralized approach to this issue could result in better care at lower costs and many more lives saved.

The reforms at the Veterans' Administration are one example. Our great veterans are now being given a choice in doctors, allowing them to escape the maddening and inefficient bureaucracy of the VA to receive care from private physicians on a timely basis.

Likewise, the Department of Health and Human Services under President Trump granted waiver after waiver to the states to give Medicaid patients more choices in health care. Association health insurance was encouraged by executive order and the direct primary care model was looked on more favorably.

Perhaps one of the most exciting developments was the President's signature on the Right to Try Act of 2018.

Formally known as the "Trickett Wendler, Frank Mongiello, Jordan McLinn, and Matthew Bellina Right to Try Act of 2018," this legislation amended existing federal law to permit certain unapproved, experimental drugs to be administered to terminally ill patients who have exhausted all other approved treatment options and are unable to participate in clinical drug trials. These drugs are not snake oil cures; they all must have completed an FDA-approved Phase I clinical trial and be in an active clinical trial as well as being in ongoing active development or production.

For years prior to the passage of the "Right to Try" Act, thousands of Americans were forced to go abroad in search of possible life-saving treatments for terminal illnesses. The Food and Drug Administration – which was created for the purpose of ensuring that only safe drugs and medications enter the U.S. market – has too often been a burdensome obstacle in the way of fast-tracking life-saving medications. Like most government bureaucracies, the FDA has constructed a byzantine complex of regulations and compliance costs that result in long delays in drug approval and massively increased research costs in health care.

The foot-dragging on the part of the FDA became even more serious after 1962, as a result of the Kefauver-Harris legislation, which dramatically increased the agency's power. Enacted as a result of some unfortunate tragedies associated mainly with two drugs (including Thalidomide), these amendments led to a steep drop in the number of new drugs entering the market each year. The reason for the decline was due to the hugely expensive and restrictive regulations imposed on the pharmaceutical companies, causing research and development costs to soar. Thanks to FDA regulations over the last half-century, the United States fell behind the rest of the world in gaining access to important medications. It is estimated that if we were to calculate the number of premature deaths caused by drug delays, deaths due to loss of innovation, and deaths due to the FDA's suppression of life-saving information, nearly half of the people who have died since 1962 had their lives shortened by eleven years.

Just the application process alone can take up to 100 hours, according to the FDA's own estimates. If you are dying, 100 hours is a lifetime and you can't wait!

As a physician who faces life and death decisions every day and whose wife is battling Stage IV breast cancer, I am angered by the FDA's policies. It is one thing to prevent dangerous, adulterated drugs from flooding the American market. It is something else to prolong the approval process to the point that terminally ill patients actually die or are forced to go overseas where these drugs have existed safely for years. And no one can say that the FDA has had a perfect record in protecting American consumers. In 1999, the agency approved a drug called Vioxx, which wound up killing 60,000 people and triggered 140,000 heart attacks. The agency has also looked the other way as cheap generics manufactured in highly questionable drug factories in China and India are permitted to enter the U.S. market.

With the "Right to Try" legislation, however, Congress and the Trump Administration made an end-run around the red-tape bureaucrats at the FDA. We know of some of our fellow citizens who have already benefited.

Bloomberg News reported in January that a California man diagnosed with glioblastoma, a type of brain cancer that is usually fatal within two years, had been granted access to a therapy called Gliovac, produced by a Belgian pharmaceutical. This individual is one of approximately two dozen or so people currently taking Gliovac. He is paying nothing for the drug and there have been no side effects in the trial so far.

In another case, Matt Bellina – a former Navy pilot who suffers from ALS (also known as Lou Gehrig's Disease) and one of the individuals the law was named for – has been receiving the experimental therapy NurOwn, which is in phase III clinical trials.

Prior to "Right to Try," the process for obtaining experimental drugs was so challenging that fewer than 1,000 people sought and received federal approval to take such drugs in 2013. That led to similar legislation being enacted in forty states over the last several years, with bipartisan support. President Trump's signature to the federal law was a crowning achievement in what has been a long overdue gift to the terminally ill.

Today, we stand at the leading edge of the most dramatic and exciting technological and research breakthroughs in the history of science and medicine. Immunotherapies and other promising treatments are offering a realistic vision – in the near future — of a world without cancer, Alzheimer's, Parkinson's and other dreaded diseases. It's time for Big Government to get out of the way and let the scientists, researchers, and innovators do what they do best: find ways to make us live longer, healthier, and happier lives.

MEDICARE FOR ALL: JUST ANOTHER FORM OF BUREAUCRATIC CONTROL

March 19, 2019

THE LATEST HEALTH CARE "CURE-ALL" BEING advanced by the radical Left in the United States is something called "Medicare for All," a misleading title, as implementation of this scheme would essentially mean the end to the existing Medicare program for senior citizens. "Medicare for All" has a price tag pegged at more than $30 trillion, approximately $9 trillion more than our entire Gross Domestic Product. Yet, it is the latest "free" program offered by the socialist wing of the Democratic Party, embraced by the likes of Bernie Sanders, Kamala Harris, and, of course, Alexandria Ocasio-Cortez, the newly-crowned Child-Queen of America's Far Left.

Now, have you or a loved one ever been refused medical treatment because your insurance company refused to pay? Would you feel any better if it was a government bureaucrat refusing to pay for your treatment, instead of an insurance company executive? Of course not. Yet, this is the alternative that the misguided advocates of "Medicare for All" health care are offering Americans. The argument that government will never refuse necessary medical treatment is belied by the fact that in nations that practice "socialized medicine," treatments are either refused or intermi-nably delayed all the time. That's why thousands of individuals flee the twin disasters of the National Health Service in the United Kingdom and Medicare in Canada to come to the United States for important medical procedures and surgeries. Have you heard of anyone leaving the United States to go to Canada for heart sur-gery or the UK for hip surgery? Not exactly.

The fact is that the "Medicare for all" model is just another form of bureaucratic control, substituting government interference in critical medical decisions for insurance company interference. Such systems are forced by necessity to work within restric-tive "global budgets," meaning care must be carefully rationed. Does Grandma really need that pacemaker or will it only delay her passing by a year or two? Government will decide that, not Grandma or Grandpa or the kids, and if the bureaucracy decides the money for the pacemaker is better spent elsewhere, guess what? The kids and grandkids better start preparing for funeral costs instead.

This "single-payer" scheme has been tried in the United States already. In Bernie Sanders' Vermont. What happened? It collapsed once the politicians realized that there was no way to pay for it without destroying the economy and driving doctors out of their profession.

Of course, the advocates of this government-managed approach to health care still like to point to Canada as a suc-cess story. However, the Canadian success story is largely a myth. Their system works well if you never get sick or require surgery. As already noted, thousands of Canadians flee to their "safe-ty-valve" neighbor to the south — the United States— where they can get the treatment they need without being placed on a waiting list for months or years. As Candice Malcolm writes in *National Review,* "In Canada, the government determines what procedures are medically necessary. Bureaucrats, not doctors, decide which procedures and treatments are covered under the CHA (Canada Health Act) – based on data and statistics rather than the needs of patients."

Other advocates of "single-payer" point to our existing Medicare program as a shining example of a system that works. Yet, Medicare really isn't even "single-payer," as 86 percent of its beneficiaries must enroll in supplemental or private "Medigap" policies to cover what Medicare doesn't. And, when was the last time you looked at the financial condition of this program? $60 billion per year (10 percent of its total budget) is being lost to waste, fraud, and abuse and the Hospital Insurance Trust Fund will be insolvent in just seven years!

And, let's consider the impact of the current Medicare program on doctors. Physicians are getting about the same reimbursements from Medicare that they received twenty years ago. Many can no longer afford to care for Medicare patients and are forced instead to take more patients covered by private insurance where the reimbursements are somewhat more generous. What will happen if it becomes "Medicare for All" with doctors receiving the same puny reimbursements for *all* their patients, young and old alike? They won't be able to stay in their profession and will abandon their practices altogether, leading to what socialism *always* leads to – shortages. Remember, most doctors aren't rich. We make a fraction of what the CEOs of big companies make, and we have to pay for all sorts of things they don't, like medical malpractice insurance and medical school loans. We are like most members of the middle class over the last couple of decades, working more and more hours for less and less money. And, we still have mortgages to pay for and food to put on the table.

America's health care system has already been poisoned enough by socialism. The massive increase in health care costs began in the mid-1960s when the socialist concepts of Medicare and Medicaid became law. We don't need to turn the entire system over to government bureaucrats, denying Americans *any* choices whatsoever, whether it be private insurance provided by employers, HSAs, or cash-only direct primary care provider practices. Americans whose health care needs are as many and varied as the images in a kaleidoscope don't need to be forced into a "one-size fits all" medical straitjacket designed by Alexandria Ocasio-Cortez.

Instead of more centralized planning, bureaucratic control, price fixing, and a deteriorating quality of care, why not give Americans back control of their own health care, free to choose what they want and need, in consultation with their trusted physicians? To paraphrase Ronald Reagan, maybe when we get the government and insurance companies out of health care, we can get the doctors and patients back in.

EMPLOYER HEALTH INSURANCE: AN IDEA WHOSE TIME HAS PASSED

April 24, 2019

HALF OF ALL AMERICANS CURRENTLY RECEIVE THEIR health insurance coverage from their employer. That figure has declined from approximately two-thirds back in 2000. For most of our history, health insurance was divorced from work. In fact, health insurance really didn't exist at all, except for some companies that began selling accident insurance in the mid-19th century. Interestingly, it was Germany under the Iron Chancellor Otto Von Bismarck that was the first modern example of a nation introducing the concept of employer-based medical coverage in the 1880s.

This model only really gained traction in the United States during World War II, when government-enforced wage and price controls restricted the ability of businesses to increase employee pay. In a tight labor market, employers began adding a health benefit to attract workers. Unions that really supported President Truman's plan for national health care in 1945 but recognized the level of opposition (especially from the American Medical Association), signed on to expanding employer-paid health insurance as the most saleable alternative. Between 1940 and 1960, the number of Americans with some kind of health coverage increased seven-fold, from 20 million to 142 million. By 1958, 75 percent of people had some kind of insurance.

The federal government provided employers a huge incentive to provide health coverage to their workers. Employer-paid premiums (and some employee premiums) are exempt from income and payroll taxes. This tax exemption costs federal and state governments over $260 billion per year and tends to benefit middle and upper-income wage-earners.

What have been the results of our employer-based health care system, which has its roots in Bismarck's "blood and iron" socialism in Prussia? Has it increased or decreased costs? Has it enhanced choice and competition or restricted it? Is there a better way to provide affordable care to all Americans?

Since 1953 (except for a brief exception in the high-inflation late 1970s), health care costs have almost always outstripped price increases in other sectors of the U.S. economy. These costs really soared after the introduction of Medicare and Medicaid in 1965, which correlated with the rapid decline in the portion of health care expenditures borne by individuals out-of-pocket. Clearly, the shift to employer and government-paid medical care throughout the 1950s, 1960s, and 1970s led to the explosion of overall costs. Health care which represented just 5 percent of the economy when John F. Kennedy was elected in 1960 accounts for almost 20 percent today.

Isn't it obvious why this occurred? Once the consumer was divorced from the cost of his or her own medical care and those costs were shifted to employers or government, that consumer become less responsible in making cost-conscious choices about health care and providers became divorced from the normal cost-constraining demands of a competitive free market. When individuals carried the majority of responsibility for their own health care costs, they were wise consumers, shopping around for the best pricing for a medical treatment or procedure and not overutilizing services for non-essential care. Today, Americans covered by employer-paid health insurance often have not a clue as to the true cost of their care. When was the last time you priced an appendectomy or gall bladder operation? Many just shrug when they see insurance statements that indicate an 85 percent "write-off" on the cost of a medical procedure, not realizing the inflated cost is a result of a system that is no longer working to provide Americans with affordable care.

And, as premiums have soared, fewer and fewer employers are even able to provide coverage and are bailing out of that system. The percentage of people covered by their employers continues to drop.

Would we be better off without this system of health insurance? Wouldn't it be better if individuals "owned" their health insurance policy (just as they "own" their home and auto policies) and could carry it from job to job? Wouldn't it be better if individuals could choose a policy from numerous companies instead of being served one choice by their boss? Wouldn't it be better if individuals didn't have to take jobs they don't want or stay in jobs they hate to keep health insurance for their families? Wouldn't it be better if we could take that $260 billion tax deduction (largely for big business and corporations) and give it to individuals as a tax cut to help them pay for medical care or to create a high-risk pool to pay for people with pre-existing conditions, rather than dumping that cost on younger, healthy people through unaffordable premiums?

The solution is the direct-payer form of health care known as the Direct Primary Care (DPC) model, which will make affordable and quality care available to all Americans, regardless of age or income. DPC will permit you, the individual, to contract directly with a physician of your choice for a low monthly fee without the interference or approval of insurance companies or government. No more networks, no more refusal of treatments; just you and your doctor, the way it used to be and the way it ought to be again. You should be allowed to use your Health Savings Account to pay for these routine medical expenses and you should be allowed to purchase an inexpensive catastrophic insurance policy (something Obamacare outlawed for people over thirty) to cover accidents or life-threatening medical events, like cancer or a heart attack.

Employer-paid health insurance may have made sense to Herr Bismarck in 1883 Germany, but is it perhaps an idea whose time has passed in 2019 America?

REDUCING THE HIGH COST OF HEALTH CARE

June 19, 2019

THE UNITED STATES OF AMERICA CARRIES THE UNEN-
viable distinction of having the highest health care costs anywhere on the planet, eating up $4 trillion per year or 20 percent
of Gross Domestic Product (GDP). That's four times the percentage of the economy the year John F. Kennedy became president! Yet, we no longer enjoy the best health statistics on record,
being surpassed by other nations in such critical indicators as
infant mortality. And, access to care is being increasingly rationed
by insurance companies, which have usurped the role of making
life and death decisions from physicians and other health care
providers.

Can we achieve better health care while reducing costs, possibly by as much as one-third or $1 trillion (enough to pay for
President Trump's infrastructure plans)? Yes, we can. However,
it will require a fundamentally different approach than the grossly
expensive and inefficient third-party payer system we have relied
on for decades.

My "Health Care *by* the People, *for* the People" model
will guarantee access to truly affordable medical treatment at

reasonable premiums, stimulate free market competition and price transparency among providers, eliminate wasteful administrative bureaucracy, and prohibit insurers from delaying or denying necessary medical procedures.

Today, we Americans pay more and get less than almost any other industrialized, First-World nation. We pay as much as $21,000 for an MRI that could cost as little as $400. $60,000 for a gall bladder removal that could cost $3,000 at a physician-directed surgery center. On average, a routine surgery at a hospital costs ten times what it really should cost. *Cui bono?* The insurance companies and their bean counters and the hospitals with their grandiosely compensated executives. It's called skimming off the top.

"Health Care *by* the People and *for* the People" offers a three-part solution out of this nightmare.

First: the Direct Primary Care (DPC) model permits patients to access physicians for a low monthly fee for routine and preventive care: physicals, blood tests, and minor medical procedures that can be performed in a doctor's office. No deductibles, no copays, unlimited visits, and no long waiting room lines. The monthly fees may vary, but are normally in the range of $50 to $100 per month per patient. Obviously, older patients who need to see their doctor more often would be charged at the higher end of that scale and younger people at the lower end. Children are even less, sometimes as low as $20 per month. By empowering providers to treat patients more proactively, the need for ER and hospital stays is drastically reduced, as much as 70 percent or more. Medicare patients receive a $100 per month voucher to pay for the membership; Medicaid patients $50 per month. As no third-party payment would be allowed, recommended medical treatments cannot be denied by government or insurance companies.

Second: Emergency Catastrophic Coverage (ECC) is available from a private health insurance company to pay for life-threatening health events or accidents and ensure that no one is bankrupted by medical bills. ECC would cover up to two weeks of hospitalization and/or ICU care. At premiums of approximately $150 to $200 per month, most Americans will be able to afford this. Those who cannot are eligible to receive a voucher from the government to pay. Those who have the means but still refuse to purchase such coverage are ultimately responsible for that decision and the costs they incur. Health insurance companies will again be carefully confined and corralled to fulfill the original concept of their trade: protecting us from something truly cataclysmic, not a profit-maximizing racket to see how many millions CEOs can be paid and how many medical treatments can be vetoed.

Third: Americans will have National Health Care Savings Accounts, possibly paid by employers in lieu of premiums paid for employer-sponsored health insurance. That can be encouraged by repealing the federal government's $250 billion tax subsidy for work-based health insurance, freeing employees from the chains of staying in jobs they dislike just to receive the health benefits and liberating employers from the costly burden of providing and administering health insurance. The funds deposited into these accounts can be used to pay for specialist visits, pre-existing conditions, and hospitalization/ICU medical care over the two-week catastrophic coverage.

The objective of this tripartite program is to make all Americans enjoy better health care and unimpeded access at a one-third savings off the current system. Just for purposes of comparison, Medicare and Medicaid cost taxpayers over $1.226 trillion annually. Providing a $50 to $100 government voucher to each recipient to access a DPC provider would cost approximately $112 billion per year. While most Medicare and Medicaid spending is for high-cost hospitalization and specialized care, greater access to a primary care physician and basic medical procedures and services will significantly reduce the need for costly hospital care.

Imagine the cost of your entire health care plan for $200 to $300 a month. It's time for Health Care *by* the People and *for* the People now!

AMERICA'S COMING DOCTOR CRISIS: IT'S ALREADY HERE

July 2, 2019

D O YOU KNOW THAT AMERICA FACES A PHYSICIAN shortage of up to 100,000 by the year 2030, according to the American Association of American Medical Colleges?

Are you aware that the majority of physicians would not recommend medicine as a career? Almost two-thirds are pessimistic about the future of their profession and 46 percent surveyed by the Physicians Foundation plan to change careers. One doctor, Ernest Brown of Washington, D.C., says there's no "heart and soul" in medicine. "It's all commodities and profit."

A 2018 survey of over 8,000 physicians reported that 78 percent feel "burned out" and 40 percent screen positive for depression, according to the AMA. Even more alarming is the fact that one doctor commits suicide every day – the highest suicide rate of any profession. That's twenty-eight to forty per 100,000 – more than twice the rate in the general population.

These are disturbing statistics and indicative of the deeper crisis facing American health care today. A great and noble profession—perhaps the noblest of all—is clearly on the ropes. Physicians are trained to heal and cure, but, increasingly, that role is being overshadowed by government and insurance company rules, regulations, and red tape that take us away from our patients. Corporate health care – dominated by a handful of powerful and politically connected hospital chains—has replaced the traditional doctor-patient-centered practice. Doctors face countless hours buried in paperwork that heals no one and endless hours on the telephone, begging for the approval of medically necessary treatment from faceless insurance company operatives. They are working longer days and nights and because of pathetically low reimbursement rates (especially from Medicare and Medicaid) and are forced to see more patients but spend less time with them. They are saddled with huge medical school debts, the need to pay for malpractice insurance, high office rents, and bill collectors, while insurance companies and hospitals siphon away more and more of their income. Unlike nurses, they have no union to fight for their interests.

One study in the *American Journal of Emergency Medicine* found that emergency room doctors spend 43 percent of their time entering electronic records, but only 28 percent with patients. The Direct Primary Care Coalition estimates that 40 percent of all primary care revenue goes to claims processing and profit for insurance companies. It certainly isn't going to doctors, contrary to popular belief. Incredible as it may sound, the average salary for physicians doesn't break $60,000 a year until after their fifth year of practice!

The problem has become so serious that thousands of doctors are leaving or considering leaving the profession. This has worsened since the arrival of Obamacare with its mandated Electronic Health Records (EHR) requirement. With a price tag of $27 billion, the EHR mandate has resulted in many small medical practices closing up and physicians either taking early retirements or selling out to corporate medical or hospital groups to afford the cost of converting to electronic records. Doctors are literally extorted to go "paperless" by having their Medicare payments cut if they do not. Sixty-six percent of physicians say EHR has reduced the amount of time they can be with their patients.

That's just one example.

Let's take a look at the coding monstrosity. In the 1980s, Medicare imposed price controls (i.e., socialism) on doctors who treated the elderly. The controls forced us to use complicated coding classifications to submit our claims to the government. The codes were tied to a fee schedule. Hospitals were required to submit to a similar coding system. This process has not only forced doctors to try to fit round pegs into square holes, consuming vast amounts of time that could be better dedicated to patients, but it incentivized hospitals to submit as many diagnostic codes as possible to the government to increase the "Medicare payday."

Private insurers soon followed the Medicare example and imposed coding regulations on physicians. By making their income dependent on how much they could bill the insurance companies, many doctors were forced to focus an inordinate amount of time on navigating codes to generate revenue for their practices. Many medical practices actually employ coding specialists and maximizing profits from codes has become something of a cottage industry in some places.

Next, we had the rise of HMOs, PPOs, and various sorts of networks the insurance companies designed to ration care. Physicians, their staffs, and patients run in circles trying to figure out if a certain doctor or hospital is "within the network" or not, often receiving contradictory information from the insurance company and the medical provider. Often, a patient will be assured that a doctor is "in network," only to find out later that wasn't the case when a big unexpected bill arrives in the mail.

Then we have the "protocols," certain pre-determined treatment standards that often do not apply to the distinct health needs of a specific individual. Again, another example of a government-imposed "one-size fits all" approach that treats us as groups, not individuals with unique needs and requirements. Doctors can face financial retribution if they don't follow the "protocols," even if their medical judgment dictates another form of treatment. And, of course, any deviation from the "diktat" must be thoroughly documented to the appropriate health care overlord.

Facing this type of straightjacket regulatory burden imposed by government and private insurers, is it any wonder almost half of physicians nationwide are actively looking to retire still in their prime or leave the medical field altogether? A recent poll showed that two-thirds of doctors said, "government involvement is most to blame for current problems." And, once the exodus starts, the physician shortage matched with the increased demand triggered by schemes like Bernie Sanders' "Medicare for All" single-payer system (as well as health care for illegal immigrants) will lead to galloping increases in health care costs and taxes, which will make today's levels look tame by comparison. Worst of all, it will lead to rationing and long lines to see your doctor or receive a medical procedure.

The crisis of American health care is at hand. If we don't want to face a dire future of medicine without doctors, we must free physicians from the strangling octopus of government and corporate control so that we can get back to doing the job we were trained to do: healing the sick and saving lives. No government bureaucrat or insurance company executive can do that.

CAN AMERICANS TRUST THE CDC?

April 13, 2020

W HEN THE COVID-19 PANDEMIC EVENTUALLY passes (and it will), we will need to take a serious look at the Centers for Disease Control and Prevention (CDC) and its role in the crisis as well as the CDC's relationship with the World Health Organization (WHO).

In recent years, the credibility and reputation of the CDC has taken some major hits, most notably its slow response to the much more deadly Ebola panic of 2014. Despite the appallingly high death rate associated with Ebola (up to 90 percent in some cases), the CDC dragged its feet in responding to the 2014 outbreak in West Africa. The agency's initial guidelines were considered too lax and were rejected by twenty-one states which opted for more restrictive policies, like three-week mandatory quarantines on all health workers returning from West Africa. Then-Congressman Trey Gowdy of South Carolina condemned the CDC's failure to provide "accurate, timely, complete, thorough information to the public." Tom Friedan, CDC Director at the time, was widely criticized for opposing a travel ban to countries impacted by Ebola.

In addition, the CDC has been criticized by senior scientists and others for its cozy relationship with corporate interests like

Coca-Cola and allowing its recommendations on public health issues like obesity to be influenced by companies producing sugar-laden beverages.

In the current situation with COVID-19, the CDC botched testing for the virus from the get-go. It developed the test on January 21, but it didn't begin shipping out test kits to medical laboratories until February 5, and those kits proved to be largely faulty. As Robert Baird observed in the *New Yorker:*

> *Still, the three-week delay caused by the C.D.C.'s failure to get working test kits into the hands of the public-health labs came at a crucial time. In the early stages of an outbreak, contact tracing, isolation, and individual quarantines are regularly deployed to contain the spread of a disease. But these tools are useless if suspected cases of a disease cannot be tested. The void created by the C.D.C.'s faulty tests made it impossible for public-health authorities to get an accurate picture of how far and how fast the disease was spreading.*

Engaging in scare tactics and pointless hypotheticals does not raise our level of confidence with the CDC either. Claiming that as many as 214 million Americans (two-thirds of our population) *could* be infected by COVID-19 over the course of the epidemic (how long is that, weeks, months or years?) was an irresponsible and unjustifiable conjecture; 214 million Americans *could* also have their homes robbed or their wallets stolen or be in an automobile accident. Could the CDC please explain the meaning of the word *could*?

The CDC works closely with another organization that should pique the suspicion of all Americans, the so-called World Health

Organization (WHO). WHO, of course, is an organ of the United Nations, the globalist entity that sees itself as a model for a coming world government. It is dominated by nations that are violently anti-American and largely ruled by authoritarian despots.

In recent years, Communist China has been engaged in an ongoing campaign to assert greater and greater influence within the UN and its affiliated organizations. According to President Trump's trade adviser Peter Navarro, the Chinese Communists have a "broad strategy to gain control over the 15 specialized agencies of the UN. China already leads four of the UN specialized agencies while no other country leads more than one."

Throughout the COVID-19 pandemic in which Communist China's lies and deceptions aggravated and intensified the spread of the virus, WHO was acting as Beijing's main cheerleader. It praised China's handling of the outbreak, applauding its "transparency" and "leadership" and saying its actions were "making us safer." WHO refused to declare COVID-19 a global pandemic until March 11 and didn't even send an advance party to China until February 10. This despite the fact that experts believe that this virus likely started as long ago as last October.

Communist China's control over the World Health Organization runs through an individual named Tedros Adhanom Ghebreyesus, the Director-General. Tedros is a dedicated Marxist-Leninist who previously served in the Communist government of Ethiopia. While health minister of the violent and brutal Ethiopian regime, Tedros was accused of covering up three cholera outbreaks. Beijing has been a leading patron and financial angel of the despotic leaders of the so-called Ethiopian People's Revolutionary Democratic Front, with the Chinese Communists financing construction of massive infrastructure in that country, including highways, skyscrapers and a metro system. When the Ethiopia-Djibouti railway was built, the Export-Import Bank of China backed the

project with $3.3 billion in loans and 400 Chinese investment proj-
ects assessed at more than $4 billion are currently operating there.
In fact, Beijing is now funding an $80 million WHO "Center for
Disease Control" in….Ethiopia.

Can Americans feel comfortable that the public health of their
nation (to the tune of $12 billion per year) is being entrusted to
an agency that coordinates so closely with an international body
largely controlled by a puppet of Communist China? Why is the
United States shipping a half-billion dollars a year to the WHO?
Wouldn't it be better if that money were spent here at home to
expand testing and hospital facilities to prepare ourselves in the
event of another pandemic like we are now experiencing?

The Centers for Disease Control and the World Health
Organization are, in many ways, two sides of the same coin.
They are ossified governmental or quasi-governmental bureaucracies with huge budgets and leaders with inflated egos seeking
to expand their authority over ordinary people in times of crisis.
As public institutions that lack the spirit or drive of innovation that
reigns in the private sector, they confront problems in a plodding,
often politicized, manner, clinging to old protocols and policies
that don't cut it in times of urgency. That's why we again must
look to the free market to help speed us toward a rapid conclusion
to the current crisis.

BIG PHARMA: A MONSTER THAT NEEDS TO BE TAMED

April 30, 2020

MILLIONS OF PEOPLE WERE OUTRAGED IN 2015 when Turing Pharmaceuticals raised the price of a sixty-two-year-old drug considered the gold standard in the treatment of a life-threatening parasitic infection from $13.50 to $750 overnight, a 5000 percent-plus increase. Likewise, the cost of the drug cycloserine, used to treat multidrug resistant tuberculosis, jumped from $500 for thirty pills to $10,800 after its acquisition by Rodelis Therapeutics. We also learned of the soaring cost of EpiPen as well as price increases ranging from 200 percent to 500 percent for two life-saving heart treatments manufactured by Valeant of Canada, the nation that is the Promised Land to advocates of single-payer health care. In one especially notable case, Questcor Pharmaceuticals raised the price of a multiple sclerosis drug from $1,235 per vial to more than $29,000!

A House of Representatives report issued in 2014 found ten generic drugs experienced price increases just a year prior, ranging from 420 percent to more than 8,000 percent.

With Americans shelling out over $370 billion on prescription drugs each year, we need to ask ourselves why these costs are escalating beyond all reason.

There's a saying attributed to the late Congressman Jack Kemp that "if you subsidize something, you get more of it, and if you tax something, you get less of it." No truer words were ever spoken.

In 2006, the federal government added a benefit to the forty-year-old Medicare program. It was called Part D and it provided for the coverage of prescription drugs for Medicare recipients. Medicare Part D handed 56 million new customers to America's giant drug companies. With the federal government footing the bill instead of the purchaser, what happened? Well, the combined profits of the largest pharmaceuticals soared 34 percent in the first year alone, to $76.3 billion. And, in the decade ending in 2012, the eleven largest global drug companies saw an incredible $711 billion in profits. Medicare prescription drug coverage has proved extremely profitable to Big Pharma, less so to the average consumer who sees galloping cost increases for relatively routine medications. Of course, Big Pharma can charge you the taxpayers anything they want for drugs as Medicare is legally prohibited from negotiating the price of prescriptions with the government. That fact alone amounts to a massive $137 billion subsidy to the drug companies, according to the Congressional Budget Office.

We are told by Big Pharma that the true reason for these outrageous prices is the cost of research and development.

That may be partially true, but only partially. The truth is that half of the scientifically innovative drugs approved in the United States from 1998 to 2007 were developed in university and biotech labs, not by Big Pharma. The drug companies also spend nineteen times more on marketing than on R&D as they blanket our TV airwaves with ads for pills that promise instant deliverance from everything from ED to insomnia. This massive marketing campaign (something unheard of just thirty years ago) has undoubtedly resulted in thousands, if not millions, of unnecessary prescriptions being written for patients who see the ads and demand the pills from their doctors, just like children will demand the latest cereal they see advertised on television from their parents.

Have no doubt about it, the cost of advertising is built into the cost of every prescription you take.

Now, in recent years – especially since President Donald Trump focused public attention on the crisis—the role of Big Pharma in the opioid epidemic has come under greater scrutiny. Billions of dollars in profits have been recklessly made while capitalizing on the suffering of victims of chronic pain. Drugs such as Oxycontin were never intended for long-term use due to their addictive qualities. Yet, the Food and Drug Administration in league with drug makers like Purdue Pharma (owned by the Sackler family whose net worth exceeds $14 billion) conspired to flood the American market with dangerous drugs like this. And the consequences have been devastating: 183,000 Americans died from prescription opioid overdoses between 1999 and 2015. Deaths from opioid overdoses in the U.S. jumped 17 percent in 2017 from a year earlier to more than 49,000. Deaths from fentanyl surged by 45 percent.

Every day, more than 1,000 people are treated in emergency rooms for misusing prescription opioids.

Andrew Kolodny, Co-Director of the Opioid Policy Research Collaborative at Brandeis University, says the pharmaceutical industry funded a "multi-faceted campaign" that "changed the way the medical community thought about opioids and changed the culture of opioid prescribing in the United States in a way that would lead to a public health crisis." It is easy to blame physicians for prescribing these deadly drugs, but physicians don't manufacture or market them, nor do we have a say in the FDA's approval process. We have to rely on the information provided to us by the pharmaceuticals and the government regulators. In a sense, doctors have been victimized too.

Thankfully, a crackdown is in the works. Hundreds of lawsuits have been filed by state and local governments accusing major drug manufacturers and distributors like Purdue, Amerisource Bergen, Cardinal Health, and McKesson Corp of engaging in deceptive marketing and ignoring the fact that these drugs were being diverted for improper uses.

In April, the federal government charged distributor Rochester Drug Cooperative and company executives with felonies for their role in spreading the epidemic. The company has agreed to pay $20 million in fines. An Oklahoma judge ruled against Johnson & Johnson in the first trial in the U.S. seeking to hold a drug maker accountable for the irresponsible dissemination of opioids. The company has been fined $572 million with the state of Oklahoma arguing that J&J's sales practices created an oversupply of the addictive painkillers and a "public nuisance" that upended lives and would cost the state up to $17.5 billion.

To break the iron grip that Big Pharma has on our nation, a number of things need to happen.

First of all, Medicare should be allowed to negotiate the prices of prescriptions with the drug companies, just like the Department of Veterans Affairs does. On some commonly prescribed medications, Medicare pays between 64 percent and 100 percent more than the VA. Why?

Second, reform Medicare Part D so that the drug companies aren't subsidized but the seniors.

Third, permit the importation of less-expensive medications from overseas so that Big Pharma is forced to compete with nations like Canada and Mexico, where people are hardly dropping dead in the streets from adulterated drugs.

Finally, streamline and reduce the length of time the FDA requires to approve new drugs. America has the longest approval process anywhere in the world, which only increases costs and delays getting new life-saving medications on the market.

Big Pharma spends billions of dollars ($2.5 billion just in the last decade) buying the Congress. Isn't it time we demanded that our Representatives and Senators refuse to accept campaign contributions from those who have become wealthy off the unnecessary suffering and deaths of so many thousands of our fellow Americans? And shouldn't we expose those politicians who continue to do so?

THE COMING MEDICAL REVOLUTION

Jan. 14, 2021

T HE UNITED STATES IS ON THE CUSP OF A NEW MED- ical revolution, a revolution driven by new technologies unavailable a few short years ago, a realization that the high-priced model of hospital care isn't working, and an administration in Washington willing to experiment with free market solutions to the problem.

President Trump was the first chief executive in U.S. history to support innovation and real reform in our health care delivery system. From supporting the critical "Right to Try" legislation to demanding price transparency from hospitals, this administration tried to bring down the cost of health care by expanding choice and injecting desperately needed competition among providers.

"Right to Try" allowed the fast-tracking of new life-saving medications and other therapeutics to the market, improving and extending the lives of those critically ill from cancer and other deadly diseases. Price transparency is vital to ending the secret agreements between hospitals and insurance companies to hide their massive inflation of the true cost of health care, allowing people – as in any other industry – to know the price of a product before purchasing it. President Trump signed an Executive Order expanding Medicare coverage for telemedicine. This allows senior citizens to receive medical care from the comfort of their homes, without long waits to see their physician. Expanding short-term insurance policies and enabling association health care policies permits more Americans greater flexibility when it comes to determining the most cost-effective health plan for themselves and their families.

With the Internet, doctors today are less dependent on in-office visits to see their patients. Simple diagnoses of common illnesses can be made over the phone, through Facetime, Zoom, or Skype. Individuals can access online physicians by credit card and receive immediate attention. The horse-and-buggy days of scheduling visits, waiting in crowded reception lobbies, and having only a few minutes to see your provider (or perhaps just a physician assistant) are becoming a thing of the past. Concierge and direct primary care doctors will come to your home or office, if necessary. They can draw blood, run an EKG test, and utilize mobile x-ray devices, eliminating the need to go to a lab or imaging center. Many such physicians even have limited in-office pharmacies, allowing patients to pay negotiated wholesale prices for some drugs. If surgery is required, they have contracts with local outpatient surgery centers, which can perform many routine surgeries at a fraction of the cost of hospitals, sometimes 60 percent less. There are now over 5,000 physicians providing some sort of DPC care, up from less than 200 in 2005.

Even as radical Democratic progressives shout for a "single-payer" health care system, their "top-down" model is already falling apart and has been for years. Doctors are burned out and bummed out. They are leaving their profession in droves or not entering medical school at all. After all, who wants to incur hundreds of thousands of dollars of debt and devote so many years of their lives to spend most of their time arguing with insurance companies or entering data on a computer? A return to patient-centered care is truly the wave of the future.

In the new medical revolution of the coming decades, the patient will be in full control of his or her health care, not the government and not an insurance company. That patient can choose any physician he wants to see, unrestricted by insurance "networks." Physicians' prices will be posted clearly on the Internet. Instead of co-pays and deductibles, individuals can purchase a "gym-style" monthly membership, allowing them unlimited visits and access to their physician by any preferred venue, 24/7. Low-income patients or seniors will receive government vouchers to pay for their care. Patients will have easy access to their personal medical records through a phone app, making it easy to transfer from one doctor to another.

Overpriced hospital care will become obsolete as physicians will offer a greater number of procedures, now done in a hospital setting, within their own walls or within the walls of specialists or surgery centers they are contracted with. Hospitalization will be required only as a last resort, not a first choice, and with the pricing for each procedure provided up front. This will allow patients to shop around for the best deal and be assured they are getting what they pay for. No surprise bills. Insurance companies will be forced back to the outside perimeters of health care, again offering simple "catastrophic" policies instead of all-encompassing policies with outrageous premiums and deductibles that allow them to dictate the type of medical care you receive. If you have insurance, you will "own" it and carry it from job to job, just like your automobile or house insurance.

This is an exciting vision, but it is more than that. It represents the future direction of health care in America. Since the Great Society of the 1960s, it's been assumed that Big Government and Big Business can run health care in an overtly fascistic fashion.

That model has failed miserably, leading to some of the highest health care costs on the planet and no improvement in the quality of care. Bernie Sanders, Joe Biden, and AOC would double-down on this failure through a fully government-run system. However, the genie is already out of the bottle and there's no going back. The future belongs to choice, not coercion; markets, not mandates and the inexorable advance of modern technology and smart medicine will ensure that not even AOC can stop that.

HOSPITAL PRICE TRANSPARENCY: A NECESSARY FIRST STEP

March 8, 2021

W OULD YOU PURCHASE A NEW AUTOMOBILE WITHOUT knowing the price? Would you purchase a new home that way? Or would you purchase any product in the supermarket without knowing the cost? For a slim slice of America – Silicon Valley zillionaires and Hollywood celebrities – that might be possible. There are always those with so much money, the price of anything is a mere afterthought.

However, for the vast majority of people, cost is the determining factor of most life events, whether it is the cost of a new car, a possible vacation, or a college education for the high school graduate. And, indeed, the pricing mechanism is the key component of our free market economic system. That's the process by which buyers and sellers conduct transactions. That's how we determine value. It's the basis of supply and demand. When government tries to intervene by imposing price controls, it distorts the free market by artificially stimulating demand and restricting supply, thus leading to shortages plus explosive inflation when the controls are eventually lifted.

In January of 2021, a revolutionary development was set to occur in the completely cost-distorted health care market in the United States. Thanks to an Executive Order signed by President Trump in 2019, hospitals would be required to post the price schedules of more than 300 common "shoppable services" in a consumer-friendly format. These "shoppable services" are those that can be scheduled in advance by a health care consumer, such as x-rays, outpatient visits, imaging and laboratory tests, or bundled services like a caesarean delivery, including pre- and post-delivery care. They would also be required to disclose public payer-specific negotiated charges and the amount the hospital was willing to accept in cash from a patient.

The importance of this new regulation cannot be underestimated or diminished. We know that hospital care is the greatest cost-driver in American health care today. At $1.3 trillion, hospital care, provided mostly by a small number of gigantic oligopolistic chains (as a result of mergers and consolidation in the industry), gobbles up one-third of all health care dollars in the U.S. The average cost of a one-day stay in the hospital is over $4,000, with the average stay clocking in at nearly $16,000. Hospital profits are also much higher than either the insurance or pharmacy industries. It is indisputable that health care costs can never be brought to heel without addressing the cost of overpriced, inflated hospital care.

As it stands now, insurance companies and hospitals negotiate rates in secret. The consumer has little or no say in the process. That is, until after he or she receives care. That's when the so-called "Explanation of Benefits" from your insurer arrives in the mail indicating the price of the procedure, the negotiated rate with the provider and the patient's share-of-cost. Isn't it nice to be able to charge your customer anything you want for a service weeks or months later? And hospitals admit to it. Author Marty Makary, Professor of Surgery at Johns Hopkins University, relates the case of a friend who required emergency surgery but was "out-of-network" with the hospital. She was charged $60,000 for the surgery. Yet, an "in-network" patient would have been charged just $12,000 for the exact same operation. When confronted by Professor Makary, a representative of the hospital stated: "We can charge someone out-of-network as much as we want. The law says we can."

While it is certainly true that a substantial part of hospital care involves emergency and unscheduled medical procedures and treatments (such as a broken leg or heart failure) in which total costs are impossible to project in advance, many procedures are elective or non-emergency. And, for these standard procedures, the costs can vary wildly based on geography and the amount of hospital competition (or lack thereof) in the region. Delivering a baby hasn't changed a great deal through history. Yet, the cost of a C-section in San Francisco can be five times the cost in Nashville. Can someone argue with a straight face that the medical skill required to perform this very common procedure is five times more challenging in sophisticated San Francisco than in more laid-back Nashville?

We know that as medical technology continues to advance, fewer and fewer medical procedures need to take place in the super-priced hospital setting, where much of the cost sustains a bloated administrative bureaucracy. Outpatient surgery centers can perform many, if not most, common surgeries at a fraction of the cost. Physicians can also perform many tests, including labs, EKGs, and even echocardiograms, in their offices for far less than a hospital would charge. And the hospitals know it. That's why part of their growth strategy has been to capture more and more of the outpatient market and charge more for it.

Price transparency is just one small step in the campaign to reduce the cost of health care in America. But it is an important step. The hospitals and insurance companies have been fighting this proposed change almost since it was first announced. They obviously have no incentive to abandon what HHS Secretary Alex Azar calls our "shadowy system" of secret pricing and negotiated rates. It has been highly profitable to them. Yet, for employers who carry the burden of ever-increasing premiums and consumers who carry the burden of ever-increasing deductibles and co-pays, it is about time for this necessary reform. Let us hope it is just the first in a series of market-oriented reforms that put patients back in charge of their own medical care.

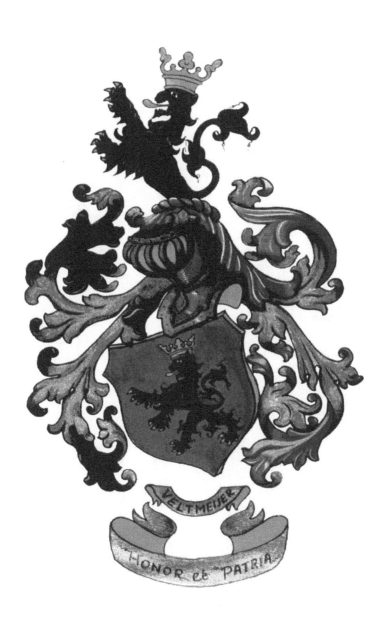

COVID-19:

A VIRAL TAKEDOWN OF DONALD TRUMP

March 12, 2020

THEY TRIED RUSSIA. THEY TRIED THE STEELE DOS-
sier. They tried emoluments. They tried the 25th Amendment.
They tried Ukraine. They tried impeachment. The globalist elites
and their handmaidens in the Democratic Party establishment
and the kept press have tried every phony trick in the book to
bring down President Trump. Yet he beat them back every time.
Somehow all of these politically inspired witch hunts and manufactured scandals were no match for a roaring economy, low
unemployment, a soaring stock market, and rising wages in the
minds of the American voter.

Of course, desperate times call for desperate measures. A
Democratic Party split between two near-octogenarian presidential candidates, one a dedicated Marxist rabble-rouser and the other
a barely coherent artifact of an arteriosclerotic political establishment, requires some kind of once-in-a-lifetime event to panic the
public and scare skittish voters into their camp. Apparently, faking
a sudden landing of Martians atop the Empire State Building
failed to materialize, so they resorted to the X-Virus, a new Black
Plague just waiting to turn American streets into modern-day

cemeteries. The X-Virus is, of course, the dreaded Coronavirus, a variant of the common cold and flu, which will be laid at the door of President Trump, lead to mass burials in major cities, crash the stock market and dump the planet into a global recession.

As a physician, I'm the last person to dismiss any new disease or virus that emerges on our doorstep. Yet, facts speak louder than mass hysteria. What we already know about the Coronavirus is that it is more contagious than the typical flu bug, but not much more deadly. With a death rate of 2 percent, it is far less deadly than SARS or MERS, for example. In fact, that death rate is likely exaggerated as many people who have been infected but have mild to no symptoms are not reporting and are not being treated. We understand that children younger than fifteen are not being affected at all. For perspective, let's consider that since 2010, between 9 and 45 million Americans have been sickened by influenza every season. The number of deaths has ranged between 12,000 and 61,000 per year.

The Asian Flu pandemic of 1957 led to 1.1 million deaths worldwide and 116,000 in the United States. The 1968 Hong Kong Flu pandemic led to between 1 and 4 million deaths globally and 34,000 in the U.S.

While the situation could certainly change, the facts as they are today do not justify waves of selling on Wall Street or hordes of shoppers trampling over each other at Costco to buy face masks and hand sanitizers. A Trump-hating media that fails to report each new case of the flu is now scrambling to scare the American people over every new occurrence of Coronavirus within our borders. In doing so, they are acting irresponsibly and reporting inaccurately, leading to the loss of trillions of dollars of wealth locked in the retirement and stock portfolios of tens of millions of middle-class Americans. They are deliberately trying to destroy confidence in the Trump economy in a despicable maneuver to trigger a recession and rig an election against the President. In so doing, the media performs its assigned role as the communications department of the Democratic National Committee, pouring gasoline on the fires already lit by the Pelosis, Schumers, and Bidens who have denounced the Trump Administration for its supposed "incompetence" in dealing with the outbreak. When the day arrives when we need to take lessons in competence from that crowd, America will already be lost.

The Centers for Disease Control aren't helping matters either, painting frightening scenarios of closed schools, churches, and massive lockdowns of all public activity. It may even recommend fallout shelters next. Of course, the CDC too is an integral part of the swamp, a bureaucratic monster whose power and budgets rise in direct correlation to how dangerous they can make a given public health crisis appear. And, what can one say about the World Health Organization, an organ of the United Nations which will look for totalitarian solutions for any emergency.

The Administration's actions to date have been sound and responsible. Restricting travel from China in the early days of the virus was something no politically correct Democrat would have done for fear of being slammed as a "racist." Let's recall that when the gruesome and far-more threatening Ebola virus reared its ugly head in 2014, President Obama refused to restrict air travel from Africa. Did we hear any complaints from CNN or MSNBC? Of course not, regardless of the danger Ebola might have posed to the American people.

What the Coronavirus has really exposed is the extent to which the United States has become dependent on a brutal communist dictatorship for so much of its manufacturing and for so many of its medical supplies and medicines. It is outrageous that innocent Americans here at home should face possible shortages of life-saving drugs because the drugs or their main ingredients are being produced in Communist China.

President Trump has been the first President in recent history to take on China and the cheap labor lobby of the Business Roundtable and the U.S. Chamber of Commerce. Through tariffs and renegotiating one-sided trade agreements, the President is providing the greatest benefit possible to the American public — redirecting the supply chains away from Beijing and back to the United States. That may lead to some temporary loss of profits for the Wizards of Wall Street, but will ultimately result in rising wages and rising living standards for the American people and a nation better able to protect itself against unexpected threats like the Coronavirus.

DO WE PERMIT A VIRUS TO DESTROY OUR ECONOMY?

March 18, 2020

A MERICA IS SHUTTING DOWN. RESTAURANTS AND bars are closing. Businesses are reducing hours. People are being laid off. Unemployment may reach Great Depression highs. Store shelves are empty. People are hoarding. The stock market has collapsed. In the short span of just a few weeks, we have descended from a high-flying economy – the envy of the world – into the abyss. We now have a small taste of what it feels like to live in a socialist nation or how things might look if Bernie Sanders becomes President.

Why has this happened? How could it happen? How could the greatest and strongest republic in the history of the world be brought to its knees by a virus that has so far infected a tiny fraction of the number of people who are sickened by influenza annually? Every year, 50,000 Americans die due to the flu or complications related to it (especially pneumonia). That's almost 4,000 people per week during a typical thirteen-week flu season. The total number of Americans who have died in the four weeks since COVID-19 became a serious public health issue: about 115 or twenty-nine per week.

Anyone old enough to recall the tragedy of polio during the 1930s, 1940s and 1950s prior to the Salk vaccine can relate stories of perfectly healthy individuals (including children) waking up one morning and being unable to walk (think of FDR at Campobello). Many recovered. Some did not.

Are we overreacting? Will tanking the U.S. economy, throwing millions of Americans out of work and bankrupting entire industries cure the virus? Will destroying our economy make it any easier for hospitals to respond to the critically ill? Will denying people paychecks and quarantining individuals in their homes help advance the cause of new antiviral drugs or a vaccine? Of course not. Certainly, social distancing and "shelter-at-home" orders might slow the spread of the disease, but at what cost? At the cost of people being unable to feed their families or pay the rent because they can't go to work? Do we kill the patient to cure the disease?

Let's get real. More than 80 percent of the people afflicted with COVID-19 will recover at home with rest, hydration and over-the-counter medications like Tylenol, many within a matter of days. Many healthy adults won't even know they have it (which raises the question, if it is so serious how come so many people will be asymptomatic?). It is true that for a small percentage of adults— mostly over sixty-five with underlying health conditions or compromised immune systems – the risk of complications, even death, rises. Why aren't we doing more to isolate the most vulnerable population in our society – our seniors – instead of those at very low risk of either infection or serious illness?

We cannot be a nation under martial law. We are a free people. We are a free nation. Forcing people to close their businesses and stay at home indefinitely is un-American and will capsize our nation, dragging down the global economy with it. Wiping out the retirement savings of tens of millions through panic on Wall Street is un-American.

Again, folks, let's get real. Too much damage has already been done and we need to step forward to mitigate any additional damage to people's lives and livelihoods.

Instead of mass quarantines, let's address the most critical issue involved in this crisis: having enough staff and resources in our local hospitals to treat those small numbers of individuals who will require life-saving intervention as a result of COVID-19. It is beyond belief that a nation that won two World Wars and conquered space cannot produce enough hospital beds and ventilators to deal with any potential flood of patients. The President's decision to invoke the Defense Production Act to greatly boost needed medical supplies makes sense, as does his action to permit doctors to work across state lines. Let's focus on the supply side of this crisis by ensuring enough medical staffing and hospital facilities to meet anticipated needs while isolating our most vulnerable populations. Otherwise, let's get America back to work.

To address the enormous damage that has been inflicted on the U.S. economy already through this pandemic of panic, let's help those who may be losing jobs or paychecks. We don't need to have the Federal Reserve engage in an orgy of money-printing to benefit the big banks, which amounts to little more than food stamps for the rich. We don't need to punish savers by embarking on zero or negative interest rates. Let's do what Germany did during the crash of 2008, help businesses meet their payrolls for workers suffering reduced hours during this crisis. Extend unemployment benefits as we have often done during recessions. Suspend estimated tax payments for businesses for the rest of the year as well as enact a payroll tax holiday. Call in the big banks and tell them to suspend mortgage payments for the rest of the year. They can afford it. We bailed them out a dozen years ago to the tune of

$850 billion and they are getting free cash every day from the Fed. It's time Wells Fargo, BofA, and Chase gave something back to their country.

Yes, we can end this crisis and we can do it soon. However, it will only get worse with permanent, long-term consequences far beyond a cough and fever if we don't ratchet down the hysteria and get our economy back on its feet now. "Flattening the curve" cannot occur at the cost of flattening our nation.

ARE WE BEING MISLED CONCERNING COVID-19 DEATHS?

March 29, 2020

A RECENT NEWSPAPER HEADLINE IN A RURAL COUNTY in Central California blared the following: "Local virus casualty was a beloved cowboy." Any reader would immediately draw the conclusion that COVID-19 killed sixty-year-old Ken Machado of San Benito County. Yet, when one reads the actual news story, this interesting nugget appears:

> *Diane Machado was careful to emphasize that county health officers who have spoken with the family said that while Ken Machado tested positive for COVID-19 after his death, that does not mean the virus itself took his life. Ken Machado had a number of existing conditions, including Lyme Disease – which he contracted about 20 years ago – and heart disease. His sister and other family members think these underlying conditions were exacerbated by the COVID-19 illness.*

Additionally, we read that the Santa Clara County Medical Examiner's Office said Mr. Machado's cause and manner of death are "pending." We also learn that the victim had undergone two major heart surgeries and retired at age forty due to Lyme Disease. He had also been in numerous significant automobile accidents prior to his death.

The tragic death of Mr. Machado raises an important question amid the panic over the pandemic. Are we receiving accurate information about the actual cause of death of individuals testing positive for COVID-19? Are health authorities and the media reporting that any deaths of individuals testing positive for the virus were directly caused by the virus? Are these reports exaggerating the true mortality numbers? Are we being misled to fan the fires of mass hysteria?

There are other examples that make us wonder if we are getting the truth. Consider this case cited by writer Christopher Ferrara:

> *A 61-year-old Warren County man who tested positive for COVID-19 died at a Lehigh Valley hospital, an advisory issued Saturday afternoon says…. Lehigh County Coroner Eric Minnich confirmed the patient died Friday night at St. Luke's University Hospital in Fountain Hill. He said the primary cause of the man's death was a head injury from a fall at home, but that the virus was listed as a contributing factor to his death. The case was one of two COVID-19 cases from Washington that were reported in the advisory. The other case is that of a 60-year-old man who is recuperating at home. They are the borough's first two reported cases of the virus.*

Italy has been especially hard-hit by the Chinese virus. More than 90,000 have been infected and more than 10,000 have perished. Yet, have all these 10,000 deaths been caused by the virus?

Apparently, the answer is no. According to Prof. Walter Ricciardi, an advisor to Italy's Minister of Health:

> *The way in which we code deaths in our country is very generous in the sense that all the people who die in hospitals with the coronavirus are deemed to be dying of the coronavirus. On re-evaluation by the National Institute of Health, only 12 per cent of death certificates have shown a direct causality from coronavirus, while 88 per cent of patients who have died have at least one pre-morbidity – many had two or three.*

In the United Kingdom, COVID-19 has been made a notifiable disease which Prof. John Lee, a former National Health Service consultant pathologist, says may be distorting the numbers of deaths. According to Lee, this means anyone testing positive for COVID-19 and later dies is being recorded on the death certificate as having died from COVID-19, contrary to usual practices for infections of this kind. He observes: "There is a big difference between COVID-19 causing death, and COVID-19 being found in someone who died of other causes....We risk being convinced that we have averted something that was never going to be as severe as we feared."

As a physician, I am on the front lines of life and death situations every day. I know that the causes of death are not necessarily cut and dry. Illnesses such as influenza can worsen existing situations in vulnerable and aging populations, but they cannot necessarily be judged as the cause of death itself. We know that as many as 60,000 deaths annually in the United States are loosely associated with the flu. Very few die of the flu itself which normally clears up in a week or two, usually sooner with an antiviral like Tamiflu. Most die of a *complication* of the flu such as pneumonia, particularly in the elderly and those with compromised lung function. This is no different with COVID-19. Consider what the CDC observed about the 2009-10 H1N1 pandemic: "It is estimated that 0.001 percent to 0.007 percent of the world's population died of respiratory complications associated with (H1N1)pdm09 virus infection during the first 12 months the virus circulated."

What we don't know is how many of the COVID-19 deaths can really be attributed to the virus or to some underlying health condition like heart or lung disease or diabetes. To truly understand the scope and seriousness of this crisis, we need accuracy. We need a denominator. We need the health establishment and media to get into the weeds of these statistics and give us the truth about what is really happening. Is this another Black Plague that will lead to the deaths of more than 2 million Americans as the doomsayers have projected or is it a more typical nasty seasonal bug whose victims may total in the tens of thousands?

Whatever it is, the Swamp is using it as an excuse in engage in the most far-reaching power grab in our nation's history. The Bill of Rights is being shredded, Americans forced into house arrest, businesses made to close, and widespread talk of martial law and troops in our streets. This is un-American, unconstitutional, and unthinkable. A $2 trillion bailout bill has been passed without even a recorded vote in the House, a bailout which will treble an annual deficit that is already $1 trillion. The Fed will add insult to injury with an orgy of $4 trillion or more in relentless money-printing, buying every kind of commercial paper in the market, with the possible exception of toilet paper. This insanity will lead to an existential crisis of roaring hyperinflation and currency debasement in the coming years, which will make toilet paper more valuable than the dollar.

As a physician, I am trained to be a healer. Right now, America needs healing more than ever before. Yes, we need to kill the virus but we also need to kill unnecessary panic and hysteria. The virus will go away, but the consequences of overreacting at a time of deep public unease and uncertainty could result in long-lasting damage to our society that far outlives COVID-19.

ARE STATE LOCKDOWNS LEGAL?

April 18, 2020

P RESIDENT DONALD TRUMP ELICITED PREDICTABLE howls of criticism – from both the left and right — with a recent claim asserting presidential supremacy over the states and their governors in the midst of the COVID-19 crisis. Suddenly, far-left governors like the radical Andrew Cuomo of New York began positioning themselves as born-again Constitutionalists and advocates of the 10th Amendment. For the Democrats whose entire political party and political philosophy is based on an all-powerful central government in Washington, D.C., to quickly pirouette into stalwart defenders of states' rights is astonishing. It is reflective of the Trump Derangement Syndrome in which anything Donald Trump is for, the afflicted must be against, and vice versa.

President Trump – rightly or wrongly – is not the first American chief executive to challenge the power of state governments. Someone named Abraham Lincoln did that 160 years ago, which led to a brutal fratricide known as the American Civil War. Lincoln refused to allow the Confederate States of America to secede from the Union, despite the fact that there was nothing in the Constitution specifically prohibiting such an action. President Eisenhower sent federal troops into Little Rock in 1957 to enforce court-ordered school desegregation. President Kennedy did the same when he nationalized the Alabama National Guard in 1963 to force Governor Wallace to allow the entry of black students to the University of Alabama. Throughout the Civil Rights Revolution of the 1960s and the busing crises of the early 1970s, numerous examples abound of the federal government – either the executive or the courts – intervening to stop state governments – especially in the South – from obstructing desegregation orders and all but seizing control of local school systems.

Today, as we battle the pandemic, governors from coast-to-coast are claiming extraordinary powers to order residents to stay home, close businesses, schools, and churches, and restrict travel and movement. People are being arrested for walking in the park, paddling alone in a river, not wearing a mask, or attending a drive-through Easter service. Is this America? And do the governors have the right to do any of this?

As Constitutional scholar Mark Levin points out, President Trump did not shut down anything. The governors did that. All the President did was issue some recommendations for mitigation and social distancing.

Power-hungry Democrats like Governor Whitmer of Michigan have behaved as authoritarian autocrats in their zeal to place their states under house arrest. How can they get away with it?

First of all, the Supreme Court long ago settled the question as to whether the federal Bill of Rights applies to the states. It does. This means that governors who continually attempt to restrict public activity may already be in violation of several Amendments of the Bill of Rights, most glaringly the First Amendment, which prohibits restrictions on speech, assembly, or freedom of religion. How about the Fifth Amendment, which prohibits taking private property for public use without just compensation? Is not the requirement to close so-called "non-essential" businesses (as determined by who exactly?) a taking of a business owner's property without reimbursing him for his lost revenue and income? Isn't jailing someone sitting alone on the beach a violation of the Fourth Amendment, which asserts "the right of the people to be secure in their persons, houses, papers, and effects, against unreasonable searches and seizures..."? Finally, how about some governors shutting down gun stores? Doesn't that infringe on Second Amendment rights, especially at a time when cities, counties, and states are releasing prisoners from jail?

Mark Levin points out that state actions to close businesses are most likely violations of the Interstate Commerce clause of the Constitution. Congress, not the states, has jurisdiction over interstate commerce. And, ever since the New Deal of the 1930s, the Supreme Court has adopted an extremely broad interpretation of federal authority over this issue. Most economic activity within a state is going to impact, in some way, economic activity and commerce in another state. Think of it this way. A restaurant in California buys meat from a meatpacker in Iowa or buys meat from a distributor within the state of California, who in turn buys it from that same meatpacker in Iowa. Closing that restaurant impacts interstate commerce! As Levin puts it:

"States have the power to regulate commerce within their boundaries, but the Congress under the federal Constitution is the only body that has the power to regulate interstate commerce. Governors, through their dictates and their fiats of what's essential and not essential, shutting down businesses — that's the ultimate regulation. If it affects interstate commerce in a very negative way, the president can in fact enforce the Interstate Commerce Clause of the Constitution, where governors do not have the power to control

interstate commerce. The state's police powers do not extend to interfering with interstate commerce. The clause was explicitly put in the federal Constitution to promote commerce nationwide."

One of the main reasons the Articles of Confederation failed in America's early years related to this very issue of interstate commerce. States were levying tariffs and other trade barriers against each other, making unity impossible. The Founding Fathers then scrapped the Articles as unworkable and ratified the Constitution instead.

Governors like Cuomo, Whitmer, and Newsom are skating on thin ice, both in a practical sense and in a Constitutional sense. They cannot lock down their states indefinitely. Constitutional rights are being violated, civil liberties are being infringed on. They are sworn to uphold those rights and liberties. It is time for them to stop playing politics with people's lives and livelihoods, stop acting like petty despots, and stop using this crisis as a way to defeat President Trump in the upcoming election. Open America now!

UNMASKING THE DANGERS OF FACE MASKS

May 18, 2020

PERHAPS ONE OF THE MOST ANNOYING – AND WHOLLY unnecessary – government-imposed mandates during the COVID-19 crisis is the increasingly widespread demand that healthy Americans wear face masks. Of course, just a few months ago, practically everyone in the elite medical establishment – from the Surgeon General to Herr Doktor Fauci, as well as the CDC and the World Health Organization – were advising *against* the use of face masks. Now, they have all shifted gears and we are being told that we must use face coverings whenever we leave our homes or enter stores. These mandates are usually being imposed by unelected and unaccountable county health directors without the approval of any elected body of lawmakers. While many law enforcement jurisdictions are refusing to enforce the mask edicts, some are and innocent individuals are being threatened with fines or jail time. And what exactly is the science behind all this?

The truth is there is no scientific evidence affirming the value of face coverings in preventing the transmission of viruses. Recent studies have been unable to establish any conclusive relationship between mask/respirator use and protection against influenza infection, according to nationally recognized neurosurgeon Dr. Russell Blaylock. While it's too early to report any studies related to COVID-19, it's unlikely masks would be any more effective against it than against the flu virus. Surgeon General Dr. Jerome Adams himself said in March that: "The data doesn't show that wearing masks in public will help people during the coronavirus pandemic."

Even the CDC in its April 13 directive only recommended the use of masks when it was difficult to maintain social distancing or in areas of significant community-based transmission. Yet, mask mandates are being imposed everywhere, regardless of any social distancing issues and even in small rural counties which have been hardly impacted by the Coronavirus. We now see perfectly healthy young adults and teenagers walking down the streets or going to the park or the beach in masks, inhaling their own CO_2 instead of fresh air. Employees of supermarkets and other chains are being forced to wear these masks all day long and are finding themselves unusually fatigued at the end of the work day. Drivers have even wound up in accidents because the masks have made them light-headed. One individual who crashed his SUV into a pole in Lincoln Park, New Jersey, on April 23, was reported by police to have fainted due to "insufficient oxygen intake/excessive carbon dioxide intake."

Dr. Blaylock cites recent studies of health care workers using N95 masks, indicating increasing episodes of headaches caused by a reduction in blood oxygenation (hypoxia) or an elevation in blood CO_2 (hypercapnia). The excessive use of N95 masks can reduce blood oxygenation by as much as 20 percent, leading to a loss of consciousness. Dr. Fauci's own National Institutes of Health reveal that inhaling high levels of carbon dioxide may be life-threatening. High levels of CO_2 are associated with headaches, vertigo, double vision, inability to concentrate, tinnitus, seizures or suffocation due to displacement of air.

And can the use of face masks actually make you more susceptible to COVID-19? The answer is yes. Dr. Blaylock observes that a drop in oxygen levels is associated with lower immunity. Hypoxia can inhibit the type of main immune cells used to fight viral infections called the CD4+T-lymphocyte. By increasing the level of a compound called hypoxia inducible factor-1 (HIF-1), which inhibits T-lymphocytes and stimulates a powerful immune inhibitor cell called the Tregs, face coverings could be setting us all up for contracting COVID-19 and other infections. Masks can also cause people to rebreathe viruses within their own bodies instead of expelling them, thus concentrating them in the lungs and nasal passages (eventually even traveling to the brain) which can even lead to the deadly "cytokine storm" that we often hear about in COVID-19 victims.

Masks are especially dangerous to cancer victims or those suffering from cardiovascular or cerebrovascular diseases, in which low levels of oxygen can promote inflammation that leads to the spread of cancers, as well as to heart attacks and strokes.

Isn't it ironic that the very face coverings that the political and medical elites in this nation want us to wear might just make us sicker and more vulnerable to a deadly second wave of the Coronavirus this fall, just about the time of the presidential election? Of course, no one could be planning something like that. That's just a silly conspiracy theory. Or is it?

For now, let's defend both our health and Fourth Amendment rights to be secure in our "persons, houses, papers, and effects..." That means that government, especially unelected bureaucrats, have no legitimate authority to force you to wear any kind of face covering in public. If the Democratic Party wants to substitute the cloth mask for the jackass as the symbol of its party, that's their business, but don't try to force the rest of us into doing it too.

ENTERING THE POST-COVID ERA

May 27, 2020

A S AMERICA ENTERS THE SUMMER MONTHS, WE WILL inevitably begin entering the post-COVID-19 era. We need to start the process of rebuilding economies, societies, and families devastated by months of lockdowns and layoffs, lost jobs and lost businesses. We have learned a great deal over the last several months, about both the virus and the response of the world's leaders to it. Much of what we have learned does not give us confidence that the actions taken to shut down our planet were justified. Has the COVID-19 crisis been another gigantic miscalculation by the global elites along the lines of the Iraq war or a more premeditated plan to usher in a new era of expanded government centralization and control, with the concomitant loss of personal liberties and individual sovereignty?

As we look back at the origins of this pandemic, our suspicions arise. We were initially assured by the so-called medical "experts" like Dr. Fauci that we had nothing to worry about. Democrat politicians like New York Mayor DeBlasio and House Speaker Pelosi were advising us to go to restaurants and bars and dance in Chinatown months after the virus had broken out in Communist China and the President had suspended air travel. We know that scientists in China and public health officials on Taiwan were warning us of the danger as early as last December. Obviously, ignoring and downplaying warnings are the right recipe for being ill-prepared in a time of crisis. Why were the medicrats and left-wing politicians downplaying a threat that they later tried to convince us was a rebirth of the Black Death? Why did the World Health Organization wait until March 11 to declare it a global pandemic? Something looks fishy about the timelines here.

Suddenly, by mid-March, everything changed. The previously dismissed Wuhan virus was now an existential threat to our very existence as a species. Chilling footage out of northern Italy reinforced the growing fear and panic. Images on the TV or computer screen are, of course, everything. Even if we're not sure where they come from or the context in which they are transmitted, they must be believed as our media masters demand. The fact that footage of Italian hospitals was carried as footage of New York hospitals doesn't matter. COVID-19 is going to get us all unless we surrender our rights to government and subject ourselves to house arrest and quasi-martial law. It is now *verboten* to go to work, attend school, run your business, or go to the beach.

Crazy models of 2.2 million dead Americans were conjured up by corrupt academicians, who themselves defied quarantine, and sold to world leaders as the result of a failure to lock down. The world's medicrats at WHO, CDC, and NIH demanded everyone submit to testing, as if testing would be any solution unless you could test all 320 million Americans or the entire world's population on a daily basis. The ubiquitous Dr. Fauci told us we might need internal passports to work, passports proving we had antibodies to the virus. Inexpensive cures like hydroxicholoroquine were ridiculed in favor of mandatory vaccines ordered by that eminent medical genius, Bill Gates.

Slowly, however, the worm began to turn. We found out that death certificates were being altered in Italy and the UK to exaggerate the number of COVID deaths. We discovered that the CDC was pressuring hospitals and physicians to list COVID as the cause of death for any respiratory issue. Seasonal flu and pneumonia cases miraculously dropped just as COVID-19 cases surged. We found out that Medicare was paying bonuses to hospitals for reporting COVID cases. We found out that 30,000 ventilators and hospital ships weren't really needed after all. Instead of overrun hospitals, hospitals began going broke for a lack of patients as doctors and nurses were furloughed. And, as testing ramped up, what happened? We started finding the necessary denominator. Millions of us had already been exposed to the Wuhan virus and didn't get sick. We had the antibodies. The true death rate plummeted to about 0.1 percent to 0.2 percent, about what is expected in a bad flu season. Doctors started speaking out that the lockdowns would inhibit "herd immunity" and spark personal health crises like alcoholism, drug abuse and domestic violence, as well as delayed "elective" surgeries, making us all sicker as a society.

Were we all snookered? Were we all taken in by the most gigantic "false flag" in world history? It's too soon to know, but huge swaths of the world's population are beginning to think so and they are making their views heard, on social media, on television, and on the streets. The People's Resistance to the lockdowns, which started as a small spark of outrage, is exploding into a full-fledged inferno of frustration, discontent, and civil disobedience. People are defying their political masters and returning to work or reopening their businesses. Some even risking jail time. Religious leaders are demanding the churches be reopened. Counties versus states. Attorney General Barr against despotic state governors. This court against that court. Lawsuits everywhere.

Where will this lead? Can we ever go back to our pre-COVID lives? Will we get our freedoms back? Will we get our country back? It's in our hands. Throughout history, governments have rarely surrendered the power they have taken from the people. It is in the nature of government to act as a cancer, constantly growing and metastasizing until it snuffs out the eternal flame of liberty. George Washington compared government to fire, "a dangerous servant and a fearful master."

Today, we face the gravest threat to our Constitutional freedoms and our national sovereignty in our 244-year history as a Republic. President Trump has referred to the Wuhan virus as the "invisible enemy." It may be that. However, we have now seen the faces of the visible enemy: Governors like Cuomo, Newsom, and Whitmer, medicrats like Dr. Fauci and Scarf Lady, and fascist technocrats like Bill Gates. They must be resisted at all costs and their power grabs and false flags exposed and rolled back in the coming months or we face a Brave New World of unimaginable tyranny and tears, a world we dare not bequeath to our children or grandchildren. As Ronald Reagan said in 1964, "We'll preserve for our children this, the last best hope of man on earth, or we'll sentence them to take the last step into a thousand years of darkness." Let it not be that last step.

THE VERDICT IS IN:
THE LOCKDOWNS DIDN'T WORK

July 22, 2020

N OW THAT THE RIOTS, LOOTING, STATUE TOPPLING, and street anarchy have subsided somewhat (perhaps due to a perception that this strategy of the Left is beginning to backfire), we're back to the left-wing media mob's screaming headlines about COVID-19. Amazingly, COVID virtually disappeared from news coverage while the mainstream media was cheering on the rioters burning down our cities and desecrating national monuments, statues, and symbols.

The current media hysterics over COVID are geared toward engineering another light-switch lockdown, as if the American economy can long survive these senseless periodic closures over a virus that still falls far short of the deaths attributed to past pandemics, like the 1957 Asian Flu.

Of course, the evidence clearly suggests that the two-month lockdown imposed on all but a handful of states between mid-March and mid-May accomplished nothing, but only made matters worse. Indeed, if the lockdowns had worked as Herr Doktor Fauci and Scarf Lady claimed, shouldn't we have largely quashed the virus and "flattened the curve" already? Why would we even be discussing new "surges" and "hot spots" at all?

Instead, we are being subjected to a new phase of sensationalism that trumpets the rise in the number of cases being reported across the country. However, what does that prove? By focusing on cases and not on deaths, recoveries, or hospitalizations, the massive increase in testing taking place would obviously result in thousands of new diagnoses. The truth is that the vast majority of reported cases involve individuals who are wholly asymptomatic, a condition that even the corrupt World Health Organization recently admitted puts them at low risk of transmitting the virus to others (the opposite of what we were told from the beginning of the pandemic and totally contradicts the logic of wearing masks).

The United States is testing more people at more times in more venues than any other nation on the planet. This testing is creating a false narrative in the mainstream media that we are in a new crisis mode and another lockdown is required. Could that have been the reason President Trump made that recent off-hand comment that there has been "too much testing"? And even the testing is itself suspect, in many instances. We are learning of individuals testing positive multiple times being reported as novel cases, and negative test results being discarded altogether.

What we need to be focused on is the fact that the death rate from COVID is plummeting. It is now lower than at any time since early March. People are recovering more quickly from the virus and there is evidence that while it continues to spread, it is becoming less and less virulent, which is epidemiologically predictable, as viruses normally weaken over time as they spread through the host population. Hospitalizations have possibly increased here and there, but some of these hospitalizations are unrelated to COVID but to the prior lockdowns, which irresponsibly and cruelly prevented elective surgeries and medical treatment for hypertension, heart disease, and cancer. Hospitals and ICUs are still not being flooded with COVID patients. In San Diego County, where I practice medicine, we have seen a fourteen-day decline in patients suspected of having the Coronavirus from ninety-eight to seventy-two, and an ICU patient decline from twenty-six to sixteen. The left-wing press likes to highlight extreme examples of individuals – especially young people — who contracted COVID and died, but usually omit any details that would give us a real understanding of what actually happened. Were any of these individuals immune-compromised? Were they drug users? Did they have other underlying health conditions? In some cases, these reports have later been exposed as "fake news."

The lockdowns didn't work. States that did not lock down, like South Dakota, have fared better than states that did lock down, like California. Nations that did not lock down, like Sweden and Japan, fared better than nations that did, like Italy. All the lockdowns accomplished was to delay the development of "herd immunity," prevent people from having their immune systems strengthened by Vitamin D, while throwing 40 million people out of work and bankrupting thousands of small businesses. There have been far greater mental health consequences to shutting down the economy and forcing people to "shelter-in-place" than the dangers of COVID-19. How about the rise of suicides and depression? How about the loneliness and despair of the elderly in nursing homes denied the ability to see their families? How about schoolchildren denied exercise and interaction with their peers by being in school?

Now, the Left is agitating to shut us down again. Governor Gavin Newsom has already done so. They see this as a way to permanently damage the economy in order to ensure a political victory for Democrats at the polls in November. Never in our history has there been a more calculated, callous, and cruel attempt to manipulate people and destroy their lives in the name of a medical crisis to achieve a political objective.

Let us emphasize once again – aside from some temporary bans on large gatherings in certain places – the country did not shut down during the Spanish Flu of 1918. Neither did we shut down in 1957 with the Asian Flu, which killed 116,000 Americans (proportionately a much lower number relative to the nation's population than the 135,000 being attributed to COVID today – which itself has been wildly inflated by including deaths caused by other maladies). We did not do so in the Hong Kong pandemic of 1968 nor with SARS or MERS either.

The American people need to take a stand now, once and for all. They need to reject the idea of any new shutdowns. They need to demand the opening of the schools. COVID-19 has been a string of lies from the very beginning, starting with the lies of the Chinese Communists to the falsehoods of Fauci and company, and the continuing disinformation scare tactics of the Trump-hating media. Enough is enough.

QUADRAMUNE FOR PREVENTING AND BEATING COVID-19

July 14, 2020

A CAVALCADE OF DISINFORMATION AND OUTRIGHT LIES surrounded the spread of COVID-19 over the last five months. Americans were subjected to numerous contradictory assertions and directives from global bureaucracies like the World Health Organization as well as the so-called medical "experts" like the CDC, the Surgeon General and the ubiquitous Dr. Anthony Fauci.

It's time to set the record straight and discuss the best ways of not just curing the coronavirus, but actually preventing it in the first place. And, as with most illnesses, it generally comes down to the immune system. Contrary to popular opinion, COVID-19 itself is not really killing anyone. What is killing a very miniscule number of coronavirus victims is the body's immune system overreacting to the presence of the virus and causing widespread inflammation of body tissues and organs, such as the lungs. Inflammation caused by the hyper-reaction of the immune system is the cause of many illnesses physicians deal with on a daily basis. Chronic diseases like lupus and arthritis are auto-immune disorders. Common allergies are caused by the immune system identifying and over-reacting to common and usually harmless outside substances (like pollen or dust) and causing that system to go into overdrive to fight the outside agent, even if that agent poses no health threat to the individual.

The reason we see most people diagnosed with COVID-19 having no symptoms or only mild illnesses is that their immune systems are functioning normally. However, in the elderly and individuals who have compromised immune systems (possibly caused by their own actions like smoking or drug use), we see the immune system moving into "freakout" mode, causing massive inflammation, often leading to either violent illness or even death.

The best defense is a good offense and vice versa. Individuals who don't want to be sickened by COVID-19 or any other viral or bacterial enemy need to strengthen their own body's self-defense capability.

With COVID-19, we know that the virus enters through lung type 2 epithelial cells. An excessive immune response results in the infiltration of inflammatory cells (neutrophils) into the lungs. Neutrophils produce enzymes that destroy the fine structures of the lung needed for respiration to occur, also causing the leakage of water into the lungs. Protection from a virus is mediated by stimulation of the first layer of defense "innate" immunity:

- interferon-alpha production
- NK cell activity
- Additional production from the virus by enhancement of Th1 cells, which are part of the adaptive immune system and cause immunological memory
- Suppression of excessive inflammation by inhibition of NLRP3 and chemicals that are toxic to lung tissue

QuadraMune is an exciting new natural health product that offers an integrated and sustained attack on inflammation. It contains four main ingredients: Pterostilbene, Epigallocatechin gallate (EGCg), Sulforaphane, and Thymoquinone. The first is used for immune stimulation and blocking inflammation. The second is a potent antioxidant, responsible for some of the health benefits of green tea. Sulforaphane is also an antioxidant and potent stimulator of endogenous detoxifying enzymes, responsible for the health benefits of broccoli. Finally, Thymoquinone is a phytochemical compound found in the plant Nigella sativa.

In a clinical trial, Pterostilbene was demonstrated to increase the ability of NK cells to kill target cancer cells. NK cells are cells of the body that directly kill viruses. In the same trial, Pterostilbene increased the production of Interferon-gamma from T cells. Interferon-gamma is essential for antiviral (Th1) immune memory. It also decreased CRP (C-reactive protein) which is associated with death from COVID-19 and TNF which is produced by macrophages in the lungs and causes lung failure.

Sulforaphane protects the lungs from damage by activating the Nrf2 gene and suppresses the death of lung cells. It stimulates production of growth factors, stimulates fluid call surfactant to clear debris, and prevents scar tissue formation.

EGCg is particularly exciting. It protects from cell death induced by inflammatory mediators, inhibits alveolar macrophage hyperactivation, suppresses neutrophil activity in the lungs, reduces fibrosis, and stimulates healing factors. It also stimulates T regulatory (Treg) cells when needed to protect the body against autoimmunity and pathological inflammation.

Lastly, Thymoquinone has an active ingredient chemically related to hydroxychloroquine, which (despite the best efforts of the left-wing press to ridicule its efficacy, has been proven in study after study to work both as a preventative and greatly assist recovery in the early stages of COVID) is demonstrated to stimulate NK cells, which are antiviral, and is a potential antiviral itself based on its mechanistic effects on cells.

Contrary to the scare tactics and sensationalistic headlines, COVID-19 is eminently beatable. Like other viruses, it can be avoided or – if contracted – its worst effects greatly mitigated by a strong and effective immune system, just like the common cold, the various strains of influenza, or other maladies that have plagued humanity for centuries. And, in this war on the virus (and any newcomers that will inevitably arrive on the scene), natural supplements like **QuadraMune** offer us real hope that the war can be won.

THE TRUTH ABOUT ANTHONY FAUCI

November 11, 2020

ANTHONY FAUCI IS THE EIGHTY-YEAR-OLD HEAD OF the National Institute of Allergy and Infectious Diseases. He has held this position since 1984. As such, he is one of Washington's most entrenched medical bureaucrats, a favorite of the political classes and media elites and whose bespectacled countenance implies a kindly, grandfatherly figure dedicated to public health and saving lives.

During the COVID-19 hysteria (which he himself contributed greatly to spreading, after previously dismissing its severity), he has become the liberal establishment's anointed high priest of American medicine, whose musings are regarded as dogma. Every word is treated as holy writ and woe to anyone who challenges his dictum.

Yet, Anthony Fauci has a proven record of being wrong – or contradicting himself – on the greatest public health challenges of our time.

During COVID, he repeatedly proclaimed throughout January and February that it posed little threat to the average American. He was opposed to President Trump's January 30 ban on air travel from Communist China, only to later retract that criticism and praise it for saving thousands of lives. He initially opposed the widespread use of masks, bolstering long-held beliefs by medical professionals that they do little or nothing to stop the spread of respiratory viruses. Later, he changed his views to demand virtually mandatory mask-wearing by Americans.

He is an advocate of large-scale and punitive Australian-style lockdowns and shutdowns, regardless of the cost to national economies, the jobs and livelihoods of individuals, or the mental and physical health of people driven to despair through drug use, alcoholism, and depression. And, he has repeatedly misled the nation about the severity of COVID-19, focusing almost exclusively on the number of reported cases, **not** on deaths or hospitalizations. He has repeatedly refused to differentiate between critical, life-threatening cases and the vast majority of cases which are asymptomatic or which resolve themselves in days with minimal treatment. He has ferociously attacked inexpensive therapeutics like hydroxychloroquine, zinc, and azithromycin in favor of highly expensive drugs like remdesivir, which is now shown in disappointing clinical trials to be only minimally effective against the virus. And, he has allied himself strongly with globalist Bill Gates (on whose "scientific" board he served from 2003 to 2010) in pushing for questionable vaccines, the risks of which are unknown.

Most seriously, however, we know that Anthony Fauci has been an open collaborator with the Chinese Communists and the Chinese Communist military in controversial – and highly dangerous – bat coronavirus research. His NIAID provided over $7 million in recent years to the Wuhan Institute of Virology to conduct these studies. It is this Wuhan Lab where some courageous Chinese scientists say coronavirus was developed and escaped from. If true, Fauci has his fingerprints all over COVID-19.

Of course, none of this is new for Anthony Fauci. At the time he took control of NIAID thirty-six years ago, the United States was in the midst of the growing AIDS epidemic. Here again, his recommendations and directives were usually wrong. He initially said AIDS could be spread casually, which we know is absolutely false and created a panic that it would soon victimize massive numbers of heterosexuals. He refused to attribute the spread of the disease to homosexual behavior, which is indisputably true, and refused to advocate for the closing of gay bathhouses. He obviously felt the bathhouses were more vital to keep open than our businesses and schools today. However, that's not surprising for a man who recommends Catholics abstain from receiving the Holy Eucharist during COVID while green-lighting strangers "hooking-up" for sex after meeting online.

In fact, during the AIDS crisis, Fauci was considered Enemy Number One by AIDS advocates. They believed that his foot-dragging on drugs and therapeutics to treat the disease was virtually criminal. As today, Fauci ridiculed therapeutics in favor of vaccines which, of course, are huge money-makers for the pharmaceutical industry. He touted a vaccine for AIDS, but it never arrived. However, AIDS advocates did see promise in an antibiotic named Bactrim, which was shown effective in preventing and treating pneumocystis pneumonia (PCP), a leading killer of AIDS patients in the late 1980s. These advocates went to Fauci and begged him to issue guidelines for physicians so that they would more readily prescribe Bactrim to treat this AIDS-related pneumonia. Fauci and his so-called "experts" refused. He said he needed "randomized controlled, blinded trial evidence." In fact, he went so far as to advocate *against* the use of Bactrim despite compelling evidence that it was working. Needless to say, his NIH refused to fund any of the trials he deemed so important, so that 17,000 people died of PCP unnecessarily. Doesn't that sound similar to his attitude on hydroxychloroquine, which has already saved the lives of many COVID patients?

If any individual in government is a candidate for term limits, it is Anthony Fauci. A career civil servant whose four decades in office have coincided with two of the greatest health emergencies in American history. And these crises only worsened on his watch. This is an individual who has likely not seen an x-ray in forty years, treated a patient, or even used a stethoscope. Yet, he is supposed to be setting U.S. health policy? A man with an unbroken record of being wrong time after time on critical life-and -death issues? Give me a break.

No, the truth about Anthony Fauci is that while he may carry a medical degree, he's no doctor in my book. I'm a doctor, I heal the sick and save lives. He doesn't. Instead, he's a denizen of the deep state, far more comfortable on the "champagne circuit" of Georgetown cocktail parties than administering oxygen in the Emergency Room. He lives for the fame and acclaim of the left-wing news media and the liberal political establishment, whose lords and ladies he extravagantly praises (check out his January 23, 2013 email in which he affirms his "love" for Crooked Hillary Clinton). He is not to be trusted with the public health of one individual in this nation and should be removed immediately from any and all positions of power and influence.

COVID:
THE GREAT DESTROYER OF LIBERTY

December 9, 2020

A T NO TIME IN RECENT WORLD HISTORY HAVE THE
nations and peoples of the planet faced a greater threat to
their God-ordained freedoms and liberties than the hyper-hyster-
ical reaction to COVID-19. To believe that this so-called health
crisis was either deliberately conceived or – at a minimum—
maliciously manipulated by the global ruling class to ignite their
"Great Reset" is to be accused of trafficking in conspiracy theories,
according to the ruling class's propaganda vehicles of the news
and social media.

Yet, we have it on the authority of Chinese scientists like Dr.
Li- Meng Yan that COVID-19 was indeed created in the Chinese
Communist Wuhan Virology Lab, funded by none other than
America's health policy czar, Anthony Fauci. Why would the
Chinese Communist Party deliberately create a virus and unleash
it on the world? Why would globalist power brokers like Fauci
fund the research? And why would the world's ruling elites choose
not to destroy the virus but the freedoms and liberties of their citizens instead?

Is it all one giant power grab aimed at frightening the world's inhabitants to surrender finally and permanently their right to travel, speak freely, practice their religion, and own private property? Why were we told back in March it was just "fifteen days" of lockdown to "slow the spread," yet those days have now become weeks and months and probably years? Hasn't Herr Fauci all but said we will be wearing masks forever and the arrival of vaccines should not change anything in our current situation of obedience and compliance?

No health crisis in recent memory has ever been addressed by rolling or "light-switch" lockdowns and shutdowns and bizarre color-coded tiers. No health crisis has been successfully brought to a conclusion through closing restaurants and private businesses. No health crisis has ever been confronted by closing churches and religious assemblies. No health crisis has ever involved closing schools. No health crisis has required mandatory mask-wearing or overnight curfews. And, whoever heard of threatening to arrest someone for entertaining too many people in his or her home?

The facts about COVID-19 could not be clearer. The virus has a survival rate of about 99.6 percent. The elderly and those with severe health issues are most seriously afflicted. Few if any children or teenagers are affected. The vast majority of individuals who test positive are asymptomatic or mildly symptomatic. There is no scientific evidence that cloth or paper masks do anything to prevent transmission of the virus. There is precious little data to suggest that asymptomatic individuals are serious spreaders of the disease. And, new therapeutics and antibody treatments like Regeneron are helping people recover faster than we could have imagined a few months ago.

Have the lockdowns and mandatory mask edicts worked? If they have, why are we having massive surges all over the country? Why are the very preventive measures Fauci and others demanded failing to turn the tide against the virus? We are masking up and socially distancing like never before, yet none of it seems to be doing any good. So, what's the response from brain-dead politicians like Joe Biden and Boris Johnson in the UK: more mandatory mask mandates and more lockdowns. Of course, it *is* the definition of insanity to do the same thing over and over again and expect a different result.

After almost a year of the progressive destruction of world society, due not to the virus, but to the response of world governments to the virus, it's time to recognize that COVID-19 is not really a health crisis at all. It's a political and politicized virus likely unleashed by the Chinese Communist Party as part of their grand strategy to weaken the West and achieve world domination, and ruthlessly used by the global ruling classes allied with the CCP to initiate the takedown of our cherished rights and freedoms.

In a stunning post-election speech by Supreme Court Justice Samuel Alito, the conservative jurist voiced alarm at what he called the "previously unimaginable restrictions on individual liberty" provoked by the pandemic. He lamented that "we have never before seen restrictions as severe, extensive and prolonged as those experienced, for most of 2020." He said COVID had become a "constitutional stress test" that "highlighted disturbing trends that were already present before the virus struck." Alito said we are moving toward a society where an "elite group of appointed experts" rules over us in the name of science.

Isn't this exactly the case where phony medical "experts" like Fauci determine public policy? And why should medical experts of any kind be determining public policy any more than economists should be making health care decisions?

Justice Alito pointed out how COVID is leading to a loss of our First Amendment freedoms across the board, from speech and assembly to religion. He said: "All sorts of things can be called an emergency or disaster of major proportions. Simply slapping on that label cannot provide the ground for abrogating our most fundamental rights."

The recent Supreme Court decision slapping down Andrew Cuomo's restrictions on church attendance in New York demonstrate that COVID – the Chinese Communist virus – has left our Constitutional rights in America hanging by a thread. By just one vote did the justices re-affirm our First Amendment rights. Four justices – including turncoat conservative John Roberts – would have flushed those rights down the toilet.

Two decades ago, we saw the George W. Bush administration launch an unprecedented attack on civil liberties in the wake of the 9/11 tragedy. That's how we got the Patriot Act, FISA, secret tribunals, and warrantless spying on American citizens. Now, we are seeing the global power brokers moving into overdrive to radically "reset" our society along authoritarian – or perhaps even totalitarian – lines. Ronald Reagan once said that if Fascism ever came to America, it would do so under the guise of Liberalism. Are we not watching that unfold today and what are we going to do about it?

IS THE COVID-19 VACCINE THE ANSWER?

December 22, 2020

I N RECENT MONTHS, BILLIONS OF DOLLARS — ONE ESTI-
mate puts the figure at over $10 billion – of taxpayer money
has been funneled into some of the world's largest corporations to
develop vaccines against COVID-19 as part of "Operation Warp
Speed." Pfizer is receiving at least $2 billion and Moderna another
$1.5 billion.

Evercore ISI pharma analyst Josh Schimmer estimates the
vaccine manufacturers will enjoy as much as $100 billion in sales
and $40 billion in post-tax profits as a result of the Wuhan virus.
For purposes of comparison, $100 billion is the total amount the
federal government spent under President Kennedy at the height
of the Cold War. Even allowing for the depreciation of the dollar,
$100 billion is still a lot of money. Author Gerald Posner has
written that "Pharmaceutical companies view Covid-19 as a once-
in-a-lifetime business opportunity."

Is this the real reason for the unprecedented rush for a vaccine
for a virus we knew very little about just nine months ago? Are
we sure the proposed vaccines will be effective or even advisable
for the vast swath of the world's population who are hardly or

even barely impacted by this virus? For example, we know children are almost never sickened by COVID-19. Do we need to be vaccinating every kindergartener on the planet or even every high school or college student? We know it is the elderly and those suffering from maladies like high blood pressure, cardiovascular disease, or diabetes who are most likely to become seriously ill from the virus. If that is indeed the case and that individuals under fifty years of age have almost a 100 percent recovery rate, why are we in such a sprint to vaccinate the entire population?

We know the flu kills hundreds of thousands of people in the world each year. Yet do we require mandatory flu shots for every individual? Of course not. A relatively small percentage of people get the flu shot and most young, healthy individuals with strong immune systems probably don't need it. The elderly and those with compromised immune systems or respiratory issues probably should get it, although it should not be mandated. And, how effective is the annual flu shot? No more than 50 percent, according to the CDC's own figures.

We are being told that Pfizer's COVID vaccine will be 95 percent effective. That means there would be a 5 percent potential rate of illness associated with it. If 300 million Americans are vaccinated, we are looking at 15 million Americans who will still possibly contract the virus. That's an enormous number of people. And, if the mortality rate of the virus is around 0.4 percent, we could see as many as 60,000 more Americans die. That roughly equals the number of Americans who die annually from the flu itself.

Now, approximately 250,000 Americans have died due to COVID, although the real figure is probably much lower, as there is a major difference in dying of COVID and dying with COVID. Many people have tested positive for the virus and died, but did not die *because* of the virus. They had other co-morbidities. In fact, in only 6 percent of cases was COVID listed as the cause of death on the death certificate. The Fake News has told us without pause that these 250,000 deaths are unacceptable. Certainly, the death of even one person is a tragedy. However, once the 5 percent ineffective vaccine works its way through the general population, will the Fake News tell us that 60,000 new deaths in vaccinated individuals is also unacceptable? We shall see.

The truth is that long before enough Americans receive the vaccine to enable "herd" immunity to develop, the virus will continue racing through society, regardless of mask-wearing and social distancing or lockdowns, all of which have just made matters worse by weakening our natural immune systems and preventing such "herd" immunity taking hold sooner, as with other illnesses in previous years. The Orwellian-like containment policies enacted by tyrannical governors like Cuomo, Whitmer, and Newsom have only served to drive the virus temporarily underground, not quash it. Once the restrictions are lifted, the virus continues to surge, which results in a new series of destructive lockdowns. It's a vicious circle.

We also know that millions of Americans will refuse to take the vaccine, for a variety of reasons. Democrats may resist taking what their leaders label a "Trump vaccine," while others will object due to ethical and religious reasons involving the use of cell lines from aborted babies. Still others are naturally suspicious of government power and government medicine and many simply do not feel threatened by COVID. In addition, the often-serious side effects (including deadly anaphylaxis and Bell's Palsy, according to one report out of the UK) with the vaccine, which can go on for days, are almost certain to dissuade people from signing up. In some cases, two doses will be necessary, and many won't return for the second batch if they are sickened for days from the side effects of the first dose.

Of course, totalitarian Democrats like the nutty mayor of Chicago, Lori Lightfoot, insist the vaccine be forced on everyone. Any kind of mandatory vaccination policy introduced by the federal government would be Hitlerian and blatantly unconstitutional – if indeed the Constitution still functions in today's America. Such a jackbooted approach to public health would undoubtedly provoke a bloody backlash among Americans already worn down and often devastated by lockdowns that have closed their businesses, churches, and schools. If there should be any catalyst for a new Civil War, it would be any effort on the part of our ruling class in Washington to order forced COVID inoculations. It would be "lock and load" and rightly so.

The COVID vaccine or vaccines (as there will be several offered by different manufacturers) are no cure-all for the virus. And they must never be used to enforce some kind of "Great Reset" envisioned by the global elites. The better approach would have been (and still is) developing and strengthening our own natural immune systems to fight the virus, while allowing us to again interact as human beings where germs and microbes are shared between us and have been since the dawn of man, allowing our bodies to build the natural resistance to all newborn pathogens. Yes, vaccines have a place, but they are just part of the solution and must remain a voluntary one at that.

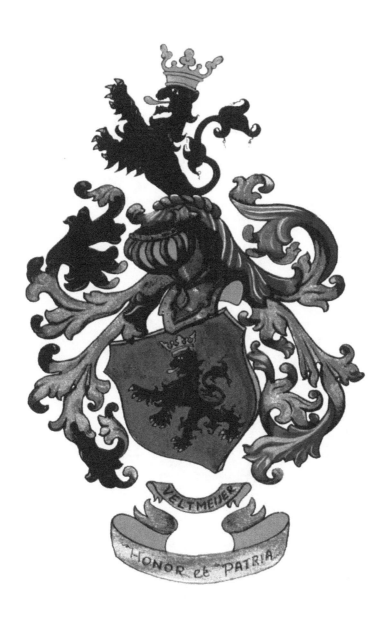

ECONOMY:

SHATTERING THE MYTH OF "FREE TRADE"

June 27, 2019

IF THERE WAS ONE ISSUE THAT DRAMATICALLY SET President Donald J. Trump apart from the corporate-political ruling class elites of both parties, it was the issue of trade. President Trump never deviated from his long-standing view that America's trade policies over the last several decades have been an unparalleled catastrophe, stripping our nation of its industrial might and manufacturing prowess, and millions of high-paying middle-class jobs in the heartland along with it.

The President was advocating fair trade as long ago as the 1980s, when U.S. trade policies were transforming Japan into such a global economic behemoth that Ronald Reagan was forced to intervene and impose quotas on Japanese cars and tariffs on motorcycles to save Harley-Davidson from extinction.

Yet, the globalist elite that controls both the Democrat and Republican parties have been addicted to the myth of "free trade" for more than half a century, dating back to 1962 when John F. Kennedy's so-called Trade Expansion Act launched the process of America's unilateral disarmament in the trade wars. At the time, the only three votes against the legislation were stalwart GOP conservatives Barry Goldwater and Strom Thurmond, as well as Prescott Bush, father and grandfather of future Presidents.

JFK's bill seemed relatively innocuous at the time, as few would see where it would eventually lead. The idea of reciprocal tariff-cutting by nations was highly appealing and Americans began enjoying the fruits of cheaper foreign imports, from Honda and Toyota automobiles to the massive assortment of inexpensive Chinese goods, from toys to clothing and shoes.

However, within a decade or so, the Trade Expansion Act's impact began being felt across the U.S. economy. Our once-huge trade surpluses with the rest of the world began shrinking and then disappearing. Foreign imports flooded the American market. Detroit was hammered as Motor City fell victim to cheap automobiles from Japan. The steel industry – once our invincible fortress in war and peace – began closing factories and shedding jobs. The textile industry was devastated. In industry after industry, the negative consequences of "free trade" were clear-cut and indisputable. Yet, American policymakers continued down their merry path of believing trade deficits didn't matter, manufacturing jobs were a thing of the past, and the future lay with corporations moving operations abroad to take advantage of lower labor costs.

Libertarians swooned to the siren song of 'free trade," arguing that nothing was more important than producing goods as inexpensively as possible *anywhere* on the planet, regardless of how many American jobs were destroyed in the process or how many American factories were shuttered.

Their views could hardly be classified as "America first."

Yet, it was President Trump's trade policies – not those of the libertarian scribblers at *Reason* magazine or the leadership of both political parties, whose donors profited off the exploitation of cheap labor overseas – that were actually in the true mainstream of American economic and political history.

All of America's Founding Fathers were dyed-in-the-wool trade protectionists, not "free traders." All embraced the Hamiltonian economic principles that sought to erect a wall of protection around the infant industries of the newly born republic. They would never have fathomed the idea of throwing open the markets of the new nation they sacrificed and died to create to the mercantilist traders of the world's empires, including the British Empire from which they had just freed us. This devotion to protectionism carried through the remainder of the 19th century and into the 20th century. Abraham Lincoln excoriated "free trade," famously saying that the difference between "free trade" and protection is that with the former "we get the goods but the foreigners get the money," while with protectionism "we get the goods and we get the money." The great pivotal election of 1896 was fought over protectionism and hard money with victory for William McKinley, who believed in a high tariff policy to protect American wage-earners against cheap foreign labor and products. His successor, Teddy Roosevelt proclaimed, "Thank God I am not a free trader."

In fact, it was the Republican Party that was historically the party of trade protectionism and restrictive immigration laws. It was the Democrats who wanted open borders and free trade.

Of course, trade protectionism got a bad rap during the Great Depression, as two chaps named Smoot and Hawley were forever condemned by libertarians for "causing" the Great Depression with their tariff bill. The truth is far more complicated than that. The fact is the stock market crash occurred months before the Smoot-Hawley tariffs were imposed and they were hardly the highest tariffs imposed in American history. And they just applied to about one-third of imports at a time when those imports only represented a meager 4 percent of our Gross Domestic Product. Herbert Hoover's huge tax increases of the early 1930s, as well as the Federal Reserve's contraction of the money supply by one-third between 1929 and 1933, had far more to do with the Depression than poor Mr. Smoot and poor Mr. Hawley.

Fast-forward to the 1990s, the decade when "free trade" went on steroids. First, we had the North American Free Trade Agreement signed by Bill Clinton in 1993. The President was correct in saying this legislation was probably the worst trade deal in U.S. history. NAFTA led to the loss of over one million U.S. jobs, a $200 billion trade deficit with Canada and Mexico, and the displacement of more than one million Mexican campesinos as well as a doubling of immigration from our southern trade partner. A year later, GATT was ratified, leading to the creation of the World Trade Organization, which surrendered Congress' Constitutional authority to regulate trade and foreign commerce to an unelected supranational body. Seven years later, the world's most predatory trader, Communist China, was ushered into the WTO. Between 2001 and 2017, 3.4 million more American jobs were lost, including 2.5 million in manufacturing and 60,000 factories closed.

And who benefited from these "free trade" agreements? Certainly not U.S. workers or their families, who saw their jobs cruelly ripped away, wages suppressed, and their living standards shredded. However, the giant global corporations profited immensely, as these agreements encouraged them to "offshore" American jobs, relocate to foreign countries, build their factories there and ship their products back into the American market, practically duty-free. It's called "outsourcing" and it is un-American and unpatriotic. To a large degree, President Trump was elected to stop this insanity that only enriches the donor class and the ruling elites at the expense of the American family.

The President's policies are working. By imposing tariffs on China, renegotiating NAFTA, and killing TPP, manufacturing jobs by the tens of thousands are returning to the United States. Factories are reopening at home as the incentive to move abroad has been removed. The American heartland, states like Ohio, Michigan, and Pennsylvania, is starting to come back to life.

We need to continue and build on these successful policies. Congressman Sean Duffy of Wisconsin has proposed the U.S. Reciprocal Trade Act, which would impose the same tariffs on foreign nations that they impose on American goods. Do you know that Communist China imposes 40 percent tariffs on U.S. automobiles and India levies a 100 percent tax on U.S. motorcycles? It is time to replace the discredited libertarian classroom theory of "free trade" with "fair trade" policies that place the interests of American workers and families ahead of the profiteering of faceless global corporations that owe allegiance to no flag, no creed, and no nation, least of all the United States of America.

THE HIDDEN HAND OF INFLATION

February 6, 2020

ANYONE ALIVE IN THE 1970s REMEMBERS WHAT WAS then called "runaway inflation." Starting in the late 1960s, the great scourge of rising prices began to grip the U.S. economy. This was the direct result of President Johnson's "guns and butter" policies, which saw the federal deficit soar, meaning the Federal Reserve System—America's secretive central bank – began printing money to lend to the government to pay its bills. Of course, printing unbacked, unredeemable paper money is the very definition of inflation. "Too much money chasing too few goods" causes prices to rise. Price increases are actually the result of inflation, not its cause, nor inflation itself.

President Nixon continued to fund LBJ's Great Society in the early 1970s while pursuing the costly war in Vietnam for another four years. Nixon's budget deficits likewise grew and a balanced federal budget was never submitted to Congress. Nixon, nervous about his own re-election in 1972, pressured the supposedly non-political Federal Reserve (hereinafter referred to simply as the "Fed") to juice the economy with funny money right before the election to ensure that he won. Fed chairman Arthur Burns complied. By the time Nixon was forced from office in August 1974, the U.S. inflation rate was 12.3 percent. That meant that prices were doubling every six years. The economy was in a shambles.

Inflation continued to be a major problem through the short-lived Ford Administration, and then raged completely out of control under Jimmy Carter in the late 1970s, hitting 13.3 percent in 1979. A major reason Ronald Reagan was elected the following year was his promise to stop the inflation inferno that was gobbling up paychecks and destroying the value of the dollar. Inflation is itself a hidden "tax," as it perniciously eats away at the salaries and incomes of the middle and working classes and seniors on fixed incomes by reducing their purchasing power. A gallon of gas that cost 25 cents in 1960 cost $1.19 twenty years later. A loaf of bread had more than doubled from 22 cents to 50 cents. A new automobile went from $2,600 to $7,200. And the price of a new house? It ballooned from $12,700 when John F. Kennedy was elected to $68,700 when Ronald Reagan prevailed in 1980.

It is said that Reagan's policies in the 1980s, which brought inflation down to 3 percent or 4 percent, broke the back of the roaring lion. Is that really true, however? How could inflation have dropped so significantly under Reagan when budget deficits had quadrupled from $50 billion a year under Jimmy Carter to $200 billion annually under his successor? Aren't federal deficits the main cause of inflation, as they require the Fed to print money to buy the government's bonds so it can spend the money it doesn't have? The answer is a little complicated, but this is my theory as to why inflation has supposedly remained tame in the low single digits for the past thirty-five years or so.

First of all, under Reagan, the United States started borrowing more money from abroad, from nations like Japan, which bought our Treasury bills. It was in the 1980s that the United States first became a debtor nation. Under previous administrations, it was usually the Fed that did the dirty work of buying the Treasury bonds with newly created money that subsequently devalued the worth of all other dollars in circulation. And, until 1971, there were some limits on that as we were still on the gold standard, at least for international transactions. If foreigners saw the Fed printing too much money, they just started redeeming their green dollars for gold bullion. This led to a virtual "run on the dollar" by the summer of 1971, when the United States had literally run out of gold to meet foreign demands. President Nixon simply "closed the gold window" in August of that year, reneging on our agreement with the world, established at Bretton Woods in 1944, that we would redeem dollars for gold at $35 an ounce.

So, by borrowing from abroad rather than from the central bank, we essentially exported our inflation. Our annual trade deficit of a mind-blowing $878 billion means we are sending all those dollars abroad, instead of them staying in the domestic economy and igniting higher inflation.

Two other major factors contributed mightily to the low inflation numbers of recent decades and they were two of President Trump's paramount issues: immigration and trade. The 1962 Trade Expansion Act and the 1965 immigration law led to the twin phenomena of cheap foreign imports flooding the United States, suppressing price increases regardless of how much money was being printed, and millions of low-wage foreign workers flooding the country, competing for jobs and stifling wage growth.

Domestic manufacturers were simply unable to pass on price increases because of the new competition from abroad. Was that a good thing? Maybe for WalMart shoppers and other "big box" consumers, but it was devastating to America's working class, which saw their automobile factories, steel plants, and textile mills shut down and their jobs eliminated. And on the labor side, throwing open the U.S. market to all comers suppressed the wages of working and middle-class Americans. Avaricious employers were only too happy to hire an illegal Mexican immigrant for $3 or $4 an hour instead of paying an American $15 or $20 an hour. Many were even hired and paid "under the table": off the books. With no mandatory E-verify in place, there was no way to validate the citizenship of any individual in this country.

Tariffs and other such trade-restrictive policies keep American producers in business and American workers employed, albeit at the cost of slightly higher prices for some consumer items. A strong border like we used to have ensured a tight labor market, enabling wages to rise without competition from legal and illegal immigrants. These are the policies America used to practice prior to the 1980s. These policies prevented politicians in Washington, D.C., from hiding their inflationary spending orgies. However, once the era of free trade and open borders arrived, the politicians could run up deficits to a trillion dollars and keep the true rate of inflation hidden and masked, at the expense of the American people, of course. We suffered the consequences of lower or stagnant wages and millions of high-paying jobs and factories wiped out or shipped to China, Mexico, Vietnam or India.

Isn't it time we stopped letting the spendaholics and central bankers in Washington cover their inflationary tracks by making Americans suffer in an endless race to the bottom, where 40 percent cannot even afford an unexpected expense of $500? We need tariffs and a tight labor market to make the American Dream again accessible to tens of millions of Americans who have lost all hope that this economy can and should work for them too.

ROLLING BACK THE REGULATORY STATE

January 6, 2020

O NE OF THE CROWNING ACHIEVEMENTS OF THE
Trump Administration is the President's successful campaign to roll back the excesses and costs of the regulatory state.

By the regulatory state, we refer to the monster of a federal
bureaucracy and its alphabet soup agencies that have suffocated
the U.S. economy through an endless stream of unnecessary rules
and regulations. Rules and regulations that have served more to
empower and enrich the bureaucrats and administrators themselves than serve any real public purpose.

When we think that when the American Republic was founded
there were just four cabinet-level departments: State, Treasury,
Justice, and War, and now we have hundreds of departments,
agencies, bureaus, and commissions imposing their mandates
and guidelines upon the American people, the mind just boggles.
Today, we have fifteen cabinet-level departments, controlling
almost every aspect of our lives, from housing and urban development to energy, education, and transportation. Many, if not most,
of these departments are constitutionally questionable at best, as

there is no authorization in the Constitution for most of these federal activities.

Let's consider how these departments have actually performed. The Department of Energy was created in 1977 and currently has a budget of $30 billion. Yet, in more than forty years of existence, DOE has failed to produce even one drop of additional energy for the nation's needs. Instead, it has only served to shackle our energy producers. President Reagan promised to abolish the Energy Department but failed to do so. President Trump should take this action and transfer the nuclear weapons responsibilities of the Department to the Department of Defense.

The Department of Education was created by President Carter as a payoff to the teachers' unions for their support in his 1976 campaign for president. Despite spending $66 billion a year, America's public schools are a national disgrace, with collapsing test scores, rampant crime, and declining academic standards. And what can we say about HUD? With $47 billion a year at its disposal, our homelessness crisis only intensifies while our largest cities are overrun by crime, drugs, and joblessness.

The *Federal Register* is that unwieldy accumulation of federal rules and regulations written by pampered Washington bureaucrats from the comfort of their cushy D.C. suites. Back in 1936, when Franklin Roosevelt was launching his New Deal revolution patterned after Mussolini's fascism, there were a mere 2,620 pages in the *Federal Register*. By the time President Obama took office in 2009, there were 68,598 pages, thirty-four times as many. Obama and his regulators had a field day during his eight years in the White House, increasing the pages in the *Federal Register* to 95,894, a jump of 40 percent by 2016.

Let's consider the cost of all these regulations to the U.S. economy and U.S. households.

According to the Competitive Enterprise Institute, federal regulations in 2016 cost American consumers and businesses almost $2 trillion, 10 percent of our GDP. If these regulations constituted a distinct country, it would be the seventh-largest economy on the planet, ranking behind India but surpassing Italy.

Federal regulations are a hidden tax passed on to U.S. households through higher prices. The cost: nearly $15,000 per household. The nearly $2 trillion in regulations actually exceeds the $1.92 trillion the IRS collected in both individual and corporate income taxes in 2016.

Now, Congress is supposed to write our nation's laws. That's what the Constitution provides for. Yet, in 2016, the 214 laws enacted by Congress were massively outstripped by the 3,853 rules issued by the regulatory bureaucracy. That's eighteen rules issued for every law constitutionally enacted by our elected representatives.

The impact on our economy has been dramatic. The Mercatus Center at George Mason University estimates that if regulations had been held just to the level they were in 1980, our economy would be at least 25 percent larger today. That's a loss of $5 trillion and about $15,000 per capita.

With his fervent commitment to economic growth and his background as a businessman who has had to deal with the dead weight of the federal bureaucracy, President Trump targeted federal regulations with one of his first Executive Orders in 2017. In his EO entitled *Reducing Regulation And Controlling Regulatory Costs,* of January 30, 2017, the President ordered that at least two old regulations be eliminated for every new one imposed. He actually did much better, repealing five old regs for every new one.

This was the most impressive effort to free the U.S. economy from the chokehold of the federal regulators since the Reagan presidency three decades prior. It went well beyond Reagan's

attempts to tame the federal dragon. According to libertarian economist Dr. David Henderson, the Trump Administration's work on
deregulation would result in raising real U.S. incomes by over
$3,000 per household. In just his first year in office, the President
succeeded in whittling down the size of the *Federal Register* by
34,000 pages over Obama's last year, an impressive reduction of
35 percent and bringing the number of pages down to the lowest
level since 1993. He also slashed the number of rules by almost
600 in one year, a 15 percent cut.

The President's deregulatory policies have sparked an amazing
rebirth of the American energy industry, leading to our nation
becoming a net exporter of energy for the first time in decades. It
has freed us from dependence on OPEC and unstable and undem-
ocratic Middle East governments. The Environmental Protection
Agency – one of Washington's most obnoxious agencies – has
been reined in. The FDA is approving more drugs—especially
generics – at a faster pace, bringing down prices and enhancing
competition. The banking system, which was largely stifled and
prevented from making loans due to Dodd-Frank, is now oper-
ating in a freer environment.

The result of these policies has been the strongest U.S.
economy in five decades with record-low unemployment, rising
wages, and steady growth. The heavy hand of government is being
swiftly lifted from the private sector and for that we can only
applaud the Trump Administration for taking on and taking down
the job-killing regulatory state.

IT'S TIME TO GET CONTROL OF FEDERAL SPENDING

January 20, 2020

EDERAL SPENDING IS OUT OF CONTROL. FEDERAL spending is completely out of control. Federal spending is completely out of control and no one seems to be concerned any-more. Fiscal sanity long ago disappeared from Washington, D.C., and both parties are responsible for it.

Let's look back at recent history. When John F. Kennedy became President in 1961, the federal government was spending about $100 billion per year. And that was for everything, from national defense to Social Security to interest on the National Debt. Even with a seemingly endless war raging in Vietnam, by the end of that decade, the federal government was still spending less than $200 billion.

Runaway inflation throughout the 1970s took its toll on the federal budget and over the next decade – even without a major war – spending had tripled. By the time Ronald Reagan was elected in 1980 – on a platform of cutting the size, scope, and cost of govern-ment, Washington was spending almost $600 billion a year. The biggest cost drivers, LBJ's enactment of Medicare and Medicaid in 1965, which put health care spending on autopilot, destroyed the free market in medicine, and created giant new entitlement programs for the middle class. In addition, Richard Nixon's decision to add cost-of-living increases to Social Security only worsened the spending crisis.

President Reagan tried, but was ultimately unsuccessful in his efforts to reduce the federal budget. Handcuffed by Democrats in Congress, along with a Federal Reserve that engineered a near-Depression through 20 percent interest rates, along with his own desire to greatly increase military outlays, spending continued its upward spike, as did deficits, which reached more than $200 billion by the mid-1980s. By the time the Gipper left the Oval Office in 1989, the federal government was spending more than $1.1 trillion annually. Only in the late 1990s, when House Republicans forced Bill Clinton to balance the budget amid a booming economy, did a small semblance of fiscal responsibility emerge in the nation's capital. The federal budget in 1999 was $1.7 trillion and for four consecutive years (1997-2001) actually ran surpluses amounting to over a half-trillion dollars.

It was under the so-called "compassionate conservative," George W. Bush, that fiscal discipline was really jettisoned. With a vice president who declared that "deficits don't matter" and a foreign policy based on reordering the map of the Middle East and launching the ruinous and expensive war in Iraq, Bush let spending soar. He also enacted the biggest expansion of the welfare state since the Great Society, with Medicare prescription drug coverage for seniors. The budget deficit doubled, spending reached $3.5 trillion and the economy collapsed in 2008. The National Debt stood at a mind-boggling $12 trillion, twelve times what it was in 1980.

Half-hearted attempts to control spending emerged after 2009, mainly through the "sequester," but GOP efforts to increase defense spending ran headlong into Democrat efforts to increase welfare spending, leading to stalemate. President Obama spent liberally as he continued or expanded the Bush wars abroad, raised taxes, and wasted billions on bank and auto bailouts and New Deal-style public works programs that did little to strengthen an overtaxed and overregulated economy. At the end of his term in 2017, we were spending almost $4.3 trillion a year, 20 percent of GDP.

Like Ronald Reagan, President Trump was elected on a platform of cutting taxes and increasing military spending. Yet, he vowed no cuts to the popular middle-class entitlement programs like Social Security and Medicare which, along with Medicaid, constitute two-thirds of all spending. These programs cannot be reduced without structural changes to the programs themselves, as they automatically kick in when a person reaches a certain age or income level. That's where the term "entitlement" comes from. And, with health care costs continuing to rise and an aging population to match, these programs are on a collision course with catastrophe. They are not sustainable as currently designed. Medicare is due to go broke in eight short years and Social Security by 2034 unless changes are made.

With federal deficits back to the post-Crash level of $1 trillion or more annually, interest on the National Debt is $479 billion at the time of this writing. That too is not sustainable. With a $23 trillion debt, if interest rates even rose to a historic average of 6 percent, we would be spending more than $1.3 trillion a year in interest, more than one out of four dollars spent by Washington. Unbelievable! Can we really expect Jay Powell at the Fed to keep interest rates artificially low forever, especially if inflation rears its ugly head?

We cannot go on forever spending beyond our means. Eventually, government will have to raise taxes to a level that will break the economy or simply have the central bank print its way out of the crisis, igniting massive inflation and destroying the value of the dollar. Is there a way out? Of course, but it won't be easy. It means taking on the sacred cows and cutting popular programs.

Should Jeff Bezos and Bill Gates really be eligible for Medicare? Do we need to be paying for their prescription drugs?

Why should illegal immigrants be receiving Medicaid?

Can we reform Social Security so that it becomes what it should have been in the beginning: an insurance program, not a welfare program, while giving younger Americans an opportunity to invest their payroll taxes elsewhere for their retirement?

Do we really need to be spending $750 billion a year on national defense (more than every other nation of the world combined) when we no longer face an imminent threat like the Soviet Empire and most of that budget goes to maintain bases in 120 countries?

Should we be paying almost a half-trillion dollars a year in interest to the money lenders, money that buys us not one ship, missile, school, or hospital? Why are we obligated to pay interest to bondholders who simply created money out of thin air to buy our debt?

These are all tough questions, but they need to be addressed. Sooner rather than later. We don't have a lot of time left and we can't keep kicking the can down the road. The calendar is closing in and the politicians in Washington better act before it's too late.

IT'S TIME FOR GENUINE TAX REFORM

April 16, 2020

AMERICA'S TAX SYSTEM IS A MESS. IT'S A HODGE-podge of thousands of rules, regulations, and laws that are constantly changing according to the whims of whichever group of politicians is in charge in Washington, D.C., on any given day. Taxes are cut, taxes are raised, new taxes are introduced, old ones are repealed, but the middle class continues to get squeezed while many giant corporations able to navigate the loopholes and special interest tax breaks wind up paying no tax at all.

Thousands of lobbyists swarm over Capitol Hill day and night, fighting for their favorite tax break, while millions of hard-working Americans struggle to make ends meet and waste countless hours filling out alphabet soup schedules and forms, attempting to make sense of the annual IRS handbook that the government won't even mail to you anymore.

In recent decades, we have seen major income tax reductions initiated by Presidents Kennedy and Reagan that led to major economic expansion. We also saw surtaxes imposed by the Johnson Administration to fund the war in Vietnam and a series of capital gains tax cuts under several administrations. Both George H.W. Bush and Bill Clinton hiked tax rates to balance the budget, only to see the resulting surpluses washed away as George W. Bush cut rates again, waged a trillion-dollar war in Iraq, and endorsed a massive increase in spending on Medicare. President Trump signed on to a large cut in corporate taxes that was long overdue, but many taxpayers felt the bite of losing their personal exemptions or state and local tax deductions.

If the purpose of taxes is to raise revenue to finance the constitutionally authorized and legitimate functions of government, we should ask: why this confusing and contradictory patchwork of deductions, exemptions, write-offs, depreciations, allowances, and constantly shifting rates on income and capital gains? Is the purpose of the tax code to raise revenue or to micromanage the economy and dole out favors for whichever special interest group has the most clout in Congress? Should the federal government be using tax law to favor one group over another in our society or to stimulate one type of economic activity over another?

Unfortunately, when government becomes as large, bloated, and overbearing as ours is, it all but invites tax code tinkering. When government starts handing out subsidies to everyone from farmers to oil companies or insists on regulating almost every aspect of economic activity, those who are taxed and regulated will hire lobbyists to fight back and demand relief or their share of the pie.

This is not the system the Framers of our Constitution intended. They never envisioned a federal government so enormous in its scope and power that a cottage industry would develop among those needing to influence public policy through the manipulation of tax law.

The Constitution itself states "No Capitation, or other **direct, Tax** shall be laid, unless in Proportion to the Census or enumeration herein before **directed** to be taken." That obviously ruled out an income tax, which was declared unconstitutional itself by the

United States Supreme Court in 1895. Only through the passage of the 16th Amendment in 1913 did the federal government gain the power to legally pick your pocket. However, the top rate at that time was only 7 percent and only applied to incomes above $500,000 ($11 million in today's dollars).

Wars are, of course, giant moneymakers for government and corporate elites. By 1918, the impact of World War I had caused income tax rates to reach an astounding 77 percent, before dropping back down to 25 percent under Republican President Calvin Coolidge in 1925. World War II sent rates skyward again two decades later, with the top rate hitting 94 percent on incomes over $200,000 ($2.5 million in today's dollars) in 1944. The top rate remained at 91 percent until the Kennedy tax cuts of the mid-1960s slashed it to 70 percent. President Reagan took it down further in 1981 to 50 percent and then to 28 percent in the 1986 tax reform. The top rate today is 37 percent. So much for the permanency of the much-heralded 1986 two bracket legislation.

Of course, prior to 1913, the federal government exercised its legitimate functions perfectly well, relying mostly on import duties and excise taxes. We had far fewer foreign wars and Washington left matters like health, education, and welfare to the states and local communities, or the private sector.

Isn't it time for a fair, just, and consistent tax system that simply raises revenues instead of providing incomes for high-priced CPAs and accountants? Isn't it time for a tax system stripped of special interest goodies? Isn't it time for a tax system that would forcibly corral the federal government within the confines of the Constitution?

The best option would be a flat tax of some kind, without any deductions or exemptions. And, hopefully without any paperwork either. A tax system that no longer taxes work or investment would be ideal. Taxing consumption rather than production would be logical and would spur rapid economic growth. We would end the practice of using taxes to redistribute wealth and instead use taxes to create wealth. The best approach I've seen is the FAIR Tax, which would do away with the federal income tax, corporate tax, capital gains tax, payroll tax, and estate and gift tax and replace them with a flat 23 percent tax on retail sales. Everyone would wind up paying, including the super-rich.

The loopholes that let Warren Buffett pay less than his secretary would be gone. The underground economy and the drug dealers would be taxed as well. Anyone who buys anything would have to pay. Some might argue that such a tax would be regressive, hitting the poor who have less discretionary income to spend and who spend a larger portion of their income on basic necessities. That argument emanates from a stubborn redistributionist mindset, but can be solved easily through some kind of a rebate paid to the neediest Americans, if necessary.

As many Americans now approach July 15th with dread and without jobs (thanks to an unnecessary economic lockdown over COVID-19), we should be asking the Trump Administration to drain the tax swamp of its lobbyists, lawyers, and CPAs and push for genuine tax reform that works for working people.

GOVERNMENT ACTION CAN'T SAVE THE ECONOMY

June 24, 2020

D UE TO THE COVID-19 CRISIS, THE FEDERAL GOV-
ernment in conjunction with the nation's privately-owned
central bank – the Federal Reserve System –flooded our economy
with trillions of dollars in new liquidity to cushion the American
people from the fallout from the completely unnecessary economic lockdown. The question we face is whether the roughly
$7 trillion in bailout and stimulus funds in the CARES Act and
in the Fed's unprecedented money-printing will actually spur a
rebirth of commercial activity or lead to another decade of slow
or non-existent growth.

The last time we tried a massive stimulus effort launched by
Washington we got the $700 billion TARP bailout of the big Wall
Street banks by the outgoing Bush Administration in 2008. That
wholly unjustified "food stamps for the rich" scheme was loudly
opposed by constitutional conservatives such as Congressman
Ron Paul and helped launch the Tea Party movement. Why should
the very banks that were responsible for the irresponsible lending
policies that caused the subprime mortgage collapse get their irre-
sponsibility rewarded by the U.S. taxpayer? The incoming Obama

Administration followed with an $800 billion "shovel-ready" stimulus plan that wound up sending money to congressional districts that did not exist and bankrupt companies like the infamous Solyndra. In addition, the Federal Reserve under Ben Bernake began a process of money-printing called Quantitative Easing which meant buying up mortgage-backed securities, Treasury notes and other paper "assets." Between 2009 and 2014, the Fed pumped $3.7 trillion into the banking system and slashed interest rates to almost zero. The result of this $5 trillion so-called "investment" directed by government planners? The slowest economic growth in decades and the worst recovery from a recession in the post-World War II era while the National Debt doubled between 2007 and 2015.

The Bush-Obama money-printing rampage was reminiscent of Franklin D. Roosevelt's clumsy efforts to end the Great Depression in the 1930s. Following and greatly expanding on the course laid down by his predecessor, Herbert Hoover, FDR tried to cure the Depression by raising taxes, massively increasing spending on phony, dead-end public works projects, paying farmers to destroy their crops amidst widespread hunger, regulating private industry in a Mussolini-like fashion, and empowering labor unions to cripple the nation with strikes. The result was no end to the Depression but another mini-Depression in 1937-38. Unemployment was almost as high as when he took office five years before. In fact, the United States had the slowest and most drawn-out recovery from the Depression than any other industrialized nation. The Federal Reserve didn't help either, by continuing to contract the money supply during this period of unparalleled economic despair. Most free-market economists agree that had Hoover and Roosevelt maintained a sound gold-based dollar and cut taxes instead of increasing them, the Depression would have been more like the 1920-21 downturn, sharp but short with a highly prosperous decade following it.

With COVID-19, we see that the politicians and central bankers in Washington, D.C., have learned nothing from history. They have no solution to *any* problem other than to spend and print money and increase debt. With the cost of the so-called CARES Act clocking in at $1.8 trillion, it is twice as expensive as the Obama plan and represents over half of all federal revenues in 2019. Of course, Democrats in Congress are demanding additional trillions in spending, including a guaranteed monthly income for all Americans, something that probably won't help the cause of getting people back to work. In addition, the Federal Reserve again slashed interest rates to zero, eliminated bank reserve require-ments and embarked on another QE of up to $125 billion *daily*. Yes, boys and girls, you heard that right, *daily*. In addition, the Fed is also lending up to $2.3 trillion to support a flagging economy. It is estimated that by the end of this year, the central bank will have created more than $3.5 trillion in new money to address COVID-19. When you add up the tab, you're looking at a staggering $7.6 trillion of spending and Fed money-printing in reaction to a virus that has proportionately claimed half the number of American lives lost in the 1957 Asian Flu pandemic. $7.6 trillion is an enor-mous amount of money. It is $3 trillion more than the entire fed-eral budget. It is more than the National Debt was in 2004 and more than our entire Gross Domestic Product in 1994.

What are the consequences of this orgy of fiscal and monetary madness? Certainly, it will make any economic recovery slower as a budget deficit that was already approaching $1 trillion will soar to $3 trillion or more. The National Debt will soon cross $25 trillion, heading inexorably toward $30 trillion, far larger than the size of our economy. It's easy for the politicians to ignore this appalling milestone as the interest on servicing the debt remains relatively low because the Fed has been engaged in a decade or more of price-fixing interest rates at artificially low or near-zero rates. That means little return for savers or investors, and less savings and less investment means fewer jobs, fewer business start-ups or expansions, and a much slower economy. And, of course, massive government borrowing crowds out the private sector from the capital markets. Most economists now agree that the days of 4 percent, 5 percent or 6 percent economic growth are behind us because massive debt and low interest rates retard new investment. We are probably now consigned to the abysmal growth rates of 1 percent or 2 percent that we experienced under Obama. We also face the ever-present danger of runaway inflation as all that new unbacked paper money injected into the economy will likely cause rising prices at some point or another. Will we wind up like Venezuela? Probably not, but it won't be pleasant either.

Wealth is not created by a federal program or a federal handout. Government has never created wealth anywhere at any time. Nor does wealth roll off a printing press or a computer entry in the banking system. Wealth is created by investment and work, by millions of producers and consumers utilizing the kind of stable money and honest pricing system only the free market can ensure. It's time that the course of nearly a century of wealth redistribution and funny money creation by our power elites be brought to an end before the American Dream is permanently lost to our children and grandchildren.

THE ARRIVAL OF "HARD" SOCIALISM

November 3, 2020

TENS OF MILLIONS OF AMERICANS TREMBLE WITH fear in anticipation of the November 3 election, and rightly so. Backed by its violent Brownshirt mobs in our streets, the Democratic Party has now become so wedded to the coercive ideology of state socialism that a victory by Joe Biden and a take-over of the U.S. Senate could easily signal the death knell of our Constitutional Republic.

Of course, the stealth forces of socialism have been surely but steadily chipping away at the foundations of our Republic for at least a century. The 1913 Wilsonian revolution led to the establish-ment of a central bank, imposition of a "heavy, graduated income tax" (words of the *Communist Manifesto*), and the repudiation of state sovereignty in favor of mass "democracy" through the direct election of U.S. Senators. These were all major stepping-stones toward the erection of a socialist state.

A central bank known as the Federal Reserve allowed money to be conjured out of thin air to finance the endless expansion of the power of the federal government.

A graduated income tax permitted the massive redistribution of wealth "from each according to his ability, to each according to his need" (words of Karl Marx).

Direct election of Senators violated the Founders' desire to check the uncontrolled passion of the mob by allowing the state legislatures to pick Senators, thus protecting the rights and interests of the states against unbridled federal power.

The advance of the socialist agenda reached new heights during the presidency of Franklin D. Roosevelt. Under FDR, the federal government essentially supplanted the role of state and local government, subordinated the private sector to the public sector and inaugurated a massive shift of power and authority to unelected bureaucrats and planners in Washington, D.C. Programs such as the National Recovery Act and the Agricultural Adjustment Act struck at the very heart of a free market economy.

FDR, who boasted that some of his best friends were Communists (and they were), even believed he could upend our Constitutional form of government by packing the Supreme Court with a handful of politically compliant appointees. Does that sound familiar?

Every administration – Democrat or Republican – since FDR has placed America on the progressive path to socialism, certainly in an economic sense, but now we face the reality of socialism infiltrating and corrupting the basic political structures of our system of government.

Medicare, farm subsidies, Social Security, yes, these are all forms of socialism as they are based on the redistribution of wealth. And, of course, socialism is based purely on coercion. Unless one is living on Gilligan's Island, socialism cannot exist without the raw police power of the state enforcing it at the point of a bayonet.

Who will voluntarily surrender his wealth and property to the state? No one. That's why the Communists killed over 100 million people to impose their corrupt and evil ideology on their captive populations. Yet, these types of programs represent a "soft" socialism of sort, vote-buying by politicians that carry an undeniable appeal to many groups of middle-class voters: farmers, senior citizens and others. As it's a "soft" form of socialism, most don't object to it because it seems like they are drawing some financial benefit, without overtly surrendering any of their liberties. Yet, all government programs take away some rights. Social Security, for example, restricts an individuals' right to 15 percent of his paycheck and the right to invest privately for his retirement.

America has now moved beyond the stage of "soft" socialism. We are heading toward "hard" socialism of the most dangerous form.

The Democratic Party and its street militias – imitating their brethren from National Socialist Germany – have rejected 250 years of our constitutional and democratic processes and believe that they can now enact their political agenda through force and violence. Their seditious mobs are unrestrained and uncontrolled, well-organized and well-trained. They will loot, burn, kill, and destroy to achieve their objectives. No American is safe from their wrath. The globalist Democrat elites have unleashed these mobs to create the "pressure from below."

The extortionist puppet-masters of the mobs are the Soroses, Pelosis, and AOCs, as well as renegade factions within the U.S. military and intelligence services. They represent the "pressure from above." We will call off the mobs and ensure your safety if you will only surrender power to us. And, if we surrender power to them, they promise the annihilation of the American way of life and the subjugation of the people to a one-party socialist state. They will abolish the Electoral College so they will have permanent control of the Presidency. They will pack the Supreme Court. They will eliminate the filibuster in the Senate. They will grant statehood to Washington, D.C., and Puerto Rico to add four Democrat Senators. The 2nd Amendment will be neutered. Yes, we will still maintain some window-dressings of "democracy," but for all intents and purposes, it will be the "democracy" of the late German "Democratic" Republic (i.e., East Germany). The Bill of Rights will be history and the U.S. Constitution subordinated to some "World Constitution" imposed by the United Nations.

At that point, "hard" socialism in the totalitarian sense will have arrived. And, once the political "restructuring" of America is implemented, your freedoms and liberties may be lost forever. Can this be stopped? It can, but only if you vote Trump-Pence on November 3.

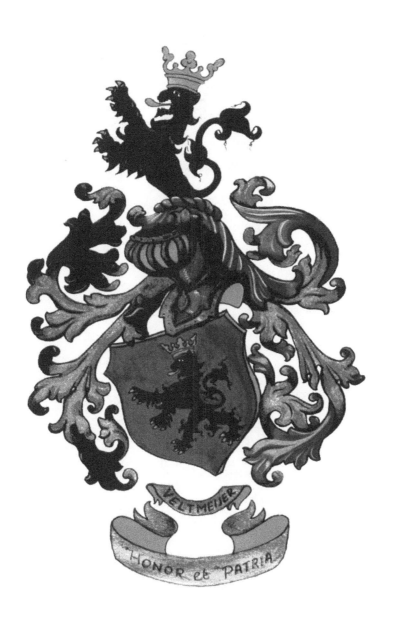

FOREIGN POLICY:

RUSSIA: THE ENEMY WE HAVE MADE

May 29, 2019

A FTER WASTING $35 MILLION AND TWO YEARS OF America's time, the so-called "Mueller Report" is in. It confirmed what we knew already and what Special Counsel Mueller probably knew as well within a few months: the entire Trump-Russia "collusion" story was a fiction. A hoax concocted by some of the most corrupt denizens of the Deep State apparatus in Washington's law enforcement and intelligence agencies, who were hellbent on engineering a silent coup to overthrow the 45th President of the United States.

While this scandal must finally be exposed, the perpetrators brought to severe justice and safeguards enacted to prevent such treasonous insurrection from ever happening again in a republic based on the rule of law, we need to focus as well on the colossal failure of American policy toward Russia since the end of the Cold War in 1989.

When the Berlin Wall crumbled in 1989 and the captive nations of Eastern and Central Europe freed themselves from forty years of Soviet tyranny and occupation, there was celebration in the West. While the Soviet Union would not technically dissolve for another three years, the genie was out of the bottle and the

127

Cold War was ending. The Red Army was going home. Ronald Reagan's policies of deterrence, economic pressure, and rolling back Communist advances in Afghanistan, Angola, Nicaragua, and elsewhere had brought the Evil Empire to its knees.

The collapse of the Soviet Empire and the withdrawal of the Red Army from Poland, Hungary, Bulgaria and the other satellite states should have heralded a new beginning in U.S.-Russian relations. Mikhail Gorbachev formally dissolved the Union of Soviet Socialist Republics at Christmas 1991. A new leader, Boris Yeltsin, took the helm of the reborn Russian nation and there was hope that democracy and the rule of law might take root in the formerly totalitarian land.

Such a new beginning should have led with a discussion of the future of the North Atlantic Treaty Organization, popularly known as NATO. NATO was formed in 1949 for the sole purpose of preventing the Soviet Union from invading Western Europe. The Soviet military alliance was called the Warsaw Pact and its control of most of the Eastern and Central European countries that FDR had surrendered to Stalin at Yalta was judged a menacing threat to the freedom of France, Germany, Britain, Italy and the other nations of Western Europe. NATO was not created to start wars, interfere in other nations' civil wars or internal affairs, or project its military assets outside of Europe. At least, that was what we were told. Thoughtful American leaders like Ohio's Senator Robert Taft were more skeptical. He believed NATO might actually provoke a new war by feeding Russia's historic paranoia about encirclement. A paranoia not without some justification. The bear had indeed been invaded throughout history, most notably by Napoleon's France in the 19th century and Hitler's Germany in the 20th century.

Now, from a logical standpoint, when the Soviet Empire imploded and the Red Army withdrew, what was the continuing justification for NATO's existence? To deter a Soviet threat that no longer existed? To confront a Red Army that was demobilized? Even Candidate Trump said NATO was "obsolete." And so it was. The failure of the West to act reciprocally and terminate that military alliance has been the main contributor to the distrust and mistrust of Moscow today, along with its own fearful military actions, meddling abroad, and other destabilizing activities.

The United States and the West had a golden opportunity to welcome Russia into the family of democratic nations in 1992 and 1993, but we blew it. Our relations with Russia since then have been a saga of broken promises, military encirclement, sanctions, and threats. Not exactly how you win friends and influence people or bring former enemies over to your side. Let's look at this sad record of the last twenty-five years:

President George H.W. Bush and Secretary of State Jim Baker made a deal with Mikhail Gorbachev in 1990. In exchange for accepting the reunification of Germany on U.S. terms, NATO would expand "not one inch" to the East. Did we keep that promise? NATO started with thirteen member states in 1949. Today, there are twenty-nine, including the old Soviet client states in Eastern Europe as well as the Baltic republics right on Russia's front porch. Even Turkey is a member.

How Turkey's membership has anything to do with preventing a Soviet invasion of Europe is a question that should be asked. The tiny state of Montenegro is a member, meaning American boys and girls are committed to fighting and dying for a country they could not find on a map. Even Ukraine and Georgia, integral parts of old Tsarist Russia, are clamoring for membership and will probably get it. Essentially, Russia is now encircled with NATO practically within its own borders. How would the U.S. feel if the old Warsaw Pact alliance was reconstituted to include Canada and Mexico and Cuba?

The old father of post-World War II "containment," George Kennan called the expansion of NATO to absorb the former Warsaw Pact countries a "tragic mistake, opining:

"It shows so little understanding of Russian history and Soviet history. Of course, there is going to be a bad reaction from Russia, and then [the NATO expanders] will say that we always told you that is how the Russians are –but this is just wrong."

The expansionist NATO—whose membership policies now resemble more of a country club than a military alliance – has also been feeling its oats since the end of the Cold War. NATO intervened in Serbia in 1999 as President Clinton led a seventy-eight-day bombing campaign on a nation that had done nothing to us, except it was a Russian ally. NATO ventured into the Afghanistan war in 2001, even though Kabul is a few miles away from Berlin. NATO continues to build up permanent land, sea, and air forces near Russian territory, along with missile defense installations in Poland. The dangling of NATO membership for Georgia and Ukraine was a leading cause of the Georgia-Russia War of 2008 as well as the crisis in Ukraine in 2014, which resulted in Russia's annexation of Crimea, a defensive move to counter continued NATO encroachment and a U.S.-supported coup against the pro-Russian government in Kiev led by President Yanukovych.

Sadly, the result of NATO's expansion has been a Russia that has turned away from democratic reforms and toward authoritarianism. The lost opportunities caused by the West's broken promises have pushed Vladimir Putin toward a revanchist foreign policy more aligned with the enemies of the United States than the potential U.S.-Russia partnership for peace Reagan and Gorbachev envisioned. The military-industrial complex that

President Eisenhower warned about could simply not tolerate the cessation of East-West hostilities, a "peace dividend" and all the rest. Their profits and power rested on perpetual war and conflict and it was relatively easy to convince naïve and gullible souls that "Russia never changes."

President Trump had a chance to change the direction of this relationship, but the Russia "collusion" hoax put an end to any hopes for that. Should he win re-election, he should follow in the steps of Ronald Reagan and develop a grand strategy to work with Russia to counter Islamic terrorism, confront China's aggressive ambitions in Asia and throughout the globe, and re-establish some sense of normalcy in relations with a country that wanted to be our friend when the Cold War ended only to be betrayed by a string of U.S. Presidents more interested in a hegemonic *"pax Americana"* than a genuine peace based on respect for national sovereignty and borders.

TOWARD A NEW REALISM IN FOREIGN POLICY

July 24, 2019

S INCE THE END OF THE COLD WAR IN THE EARLY 1990s, America's foreign policy lost the unifying theme and focus that had guided it since the end of World War II. During the post-War period, Americans enjoyed a certitude of the moral imperative of resisting communist tyranny. After 1990, our purpose seemed to shift and sway from promoting "human rights" to encouraging "democracy" to various sorts of globaloney.

This has led to a variety of misplaced priorities and policies that have resulted in staggering debacles like the wars in Afghanistan and Iraq, as well as military interventions in Serbia, Syria, Libya and other nations, costing U.S. taxpayers trillions of dollars and thousands of lives. President Trump is attempting to extricate the U.S. from some of these quicksand conflicts, only to encounter stiff resistance from the "neo-conservative" pro-war Washington establishment as well as some of his own advisors, like National Security Advisor John Bolton, an architect of the Iraq War.

After World War II, as the sole economic superpower on the planet and an aggressive Soviet Union subjugating central and eastern Europe and fomenting a communist takeover of mainland

China, leadership of the so-called "Free World" passed to the United States. For more than forty years, the U.S. – practically singlehandedly – embarked on a policy of "containment" of Soviet and Chinese communism, leading to wars in Korea, Vietnam and elsewhere.

"Containment" was the bipartisan consensus of the foreign policy establishment, rejecting grandiose concepts of actually rolling back the communist advance and liberating the enslaved nations of eastern Europe. President Eisenhower rejected calls to intervene in the Hungarian uprising of 1956. Yet, even some of these "containment" strategies were misplaced as the disastrous war in Vietnam demonstrated, radicalizing an entire generation of America's young people and almost provoking a civil war at home.

America – with its economic strength and nuclear arsenal – eventually prevailed in the Cold War, but not before President Reagan's policies forced the Soviet economy to the brink of collapse and Secretary Gorbachev to the negotiating table. Reagan, who was cautious in his use of military force, employed a clever strategy of undermining the Soviet economy while arming anti-communist rebel armies around the world to weaken and eventually bring down the Soviet Empire. Reagan wisely avoided large-scale interventions abroad.

With the fall of the Berlin Wall, the liberation of eastern and central Europe, and the dissolution of the Soviet Union itself in 1991, it was time for a new bipartisan foreign policy consensus, and one seemed to emerge, but was it the right strategy for America's third century?

With Republican President George H.W. Bush's proclamation of a "New World Order" and initiation of Operation Desert Storm in 1990, it appeared as if the direction of U.S. foreign policy would abandon the high hopes of many for a post-Cold War "peace dividend," a return to normalcy at home and abroad, and possibly a reapproachment with a non-communist Russia.

The Persian Gulf War ushered in a quarter-century of wars and military interventions around the world, often with little or no national interest involved. Was there any American interest in bombing Serbia for eighty days in 1999 under Bill Clinton? Or Clinton's prior interventions in Haiti and Somalia? How about Obama's intervention to topple Khadafy in Libya in 2011? Or the ongoing involvement in the Syrian civil war? Will the American people benefit from replacing the secular ruler Assad (who protects the religious rights of Christians) with emissaries of radical Islam?

Of course, the tragic disaster of the Iraq War represents perhaps the worst foreign policy decision since LBJ went to war in Vietnam in 1965. Fabricated on false intelligence, egged on by the "neo-conservative" talking heads like Bill Kristol, and with no clear long-term strategy, the war simply served to destabilize the entire Middle East, upset the balance of power in the region, and exacerbate the threat from Iran. Far from creating "democracies" in that part of the world, it only unleashed the profoundly anti-democratic forces of Islamic extremism and terrorism, and empowered groups like Isis.

While noble concepts like promoting "human rights," Western values, and "democracy" sound good in political speeches, they are simply not appropriate to a hard-headed, common-sense foreign policy based on dealing with the world the way it is, not as we would wish it to be. We need a foreign policy based on enlightened realism and the national interest, not high-sounding campaign rhetoric.

President Trump campaigned on a platform that shared the same vision as many of America's Founding Fathers. George Washington warned against entangling alliances with other countries and John Quincy Adams said the United States "does not go abroad in search of monsters to destroy." President Trump condemned the Iraq War and nation-building overseas. He demanded that our NATO allies as well as Japan and South Korea start paying the cost of their own defense, instead of freeloading on American taxpayers. He sought engagement and negotiation, instead of war, with Kim Jong-un. He opposed the crazy notion of war with Russia and paid dearly for it.

Unfortunately, the "neo-con" faction within the Republican Party that sees war as a 24/7 necessity, pushed back ferociously on a President who was, in his heart, a non-interventionist. They pushed him into two bombings on Syria over still unproven allegations of chemical weapons use by the Assad regime. They denounced his plans to withdraw U.S. troops from Syria and Afghanistan, apparently believing in a permanent U.S. military presence in those nations, something that only inflames native populations against us, as it did in Vietnam. They salivate for war with Iran, which would likely lead to a bigger military and political disaster than Vietnam and Iraq combined. These warmongers embody the very "military-industrial complex" that President Eisenhower warned us against in his Farewell Address in 1961. They are ready to employ every tool in their arsenal to get what they want, including staging false-flag incidents.

Winston Churchill once said it is better to "jaw, jaw than war, war," meaning it's better to try to negotiate with your adversaries and only pull the trigger as a last resort. This is what President Trump believes. Unfortunately, too many members of the foreign policy establishment yearn for a return to the Bush-Clinton years of endless military conflict. We pray that the President's vision prevails instead.

DONALD TRUMP AND ENDLESS WARS

November 2, 2019

T HE FOREIGN POLICY ESTABLISHMENT WAS UNDER-
standably enraged when President Trump announced his
intentions to withdraw U.S. military forces from Syria.

Both late last year and just recently, President Trump expressed
a determination to exit the Syrian Civil War. That determination
reflected his "America first" campaign promise to stop the endless
wars and senseless foreign adventurism of the Bush, Clinton, and
Obama administrations.

Of course, an "America first" foreign policy is the antithesis
of the globalist foreign policy of the ruling class. The globalists
seek to use U.S. military power to act as a world policeman in
advancing their objective of forging a sovereignty-dissolving one-
world government.

Donald Trump rejects such an un-American agenda. Like the
Founding Fathers of our Republic—Washington, Jefferson, and
Adams — he is a fierce defender of America's borders and sovereignty. He opposes foreign entanglements and interventions that
sacrifice our sons and daughters on distant battlefields in wars that
are none of our business.

The Middle East has been a cauldron of hate and discord for thousands of years.

Ethnic and sectarian warfare has been the rule, not the exception. Nations and empires have come and gone and come again (i.e., Israel). Unlike in past decades when the fear of Soviet intervention or the fear of losing oil supplies might have justified a U.S. military presence, these threats no longer exist. Sadat kicked the Soviet Union out of Egypt in 1973 and the Soviet Union itself disappeared in 1992. And, thanks to President Trump's policies, America is now energy independent and no longer dependent on Arab oil.

Yet, the globalists act as if nothing has changed. They yearn for the years of Poppy Bush when a "New World Order" was proclaimed at the 1991 State of the Union address. Bush, the high priest of globalism at that time, ushered in a thirty-year war in the Middle East through Operation Desert Storm.

When Iraq invaded Kuwait in the summer of 1990, few people initially saw this as a reason to start World War III. Iraq and Kuwait had long-standing border disputes and the rulers of Kuwait were hardly less odious than Saddam Hussein. Our own Ambassador April Glaspie had told Saddam just weeks before the invasion that the U.S. had no position on these Arab border disputes.

Yet, with predictable prodding from the British, George H.W. Bush decided that the fate of the planet depended on kicking Saddam out of Kuwait. After all, can you imagine how horrible it would be if the Iraqi dictator grabbed Kuwait's oil? He might just want to sell it!

So, ignoring the prescient advice of his sagacious predecessor Ronald Reagan to avoid the quicksand of the Middle East, Bush sent American boys and girls to the Middle East to save the Emir of Kuwait. The same Emir who, along with the royal family, sat out the war at the casino tables of Monte Carlo while Americans suffered and died.

Reagan, on the other hand, had refused to let himself get drawn into the Middle East quagmire. After he sent "peace-keeping" troops to Lebanon in 1983 and the subsequent bombing of the Marine barracks in Beirut cost 240 American lives, the President wisely withdrew the Marines and they never returned. While Reagan did bomb Qaddafi in Libya in 1986 in retaliation for the attack on the Berlin nightclub, the bombing was precise and targeted. No American troops entered Tripoli and there was no plan for "regime change." Qaddafi backed off and later became an ally in the war on terrorism until Barack Obama and Hillary Clinton decided it best that he be overthrown in 2011, which led to only more instability and chaos in the region.

Ever since Bush the Elder launched the Persian Gulf War in 1991, the U.S. has seen not a single day of peace in the Middle East. Throughout the 1990s – despite the fact that Saddam Hussein had invaded no other countries – the U.S. bombed that nation on a regular basis, leading to the deaths of tens of thousands of inno-cent civilians, including children. Facing impeachment in 1998, Bill Clinton launched another "Wag the Dog" attack on Baghdad.

By the late 1990s, a shadowy organization calling itself the "Project for the New American Century" emerged from the saber-rattling fever swamps of the neo-conservative underground. This outfit openly called for redrawing the entire map of the Middle East and enlisting the armed forces of the United States to engage in perpetual "regime-change" war to impose Jeffersonian democ-racies on Arab capitals. Ominously, PNAC argued that it would probably take another Pearl Harbor to mobilize American public opinion behind unending war in the Middle East.

Voila, and the tragedy of 9/11 occurred. Almost twenty years and $7 trillion dollars later, U.S. troops are still in Afghanistan (a nation that did not attack the Twin Towers on that tragic day) and Iraq, both Libya and Syria have been destabilized by civil war either initiated or aided by the Obama Administration, and the peace process between Israel and the Palestinians is all but dead. The Middle East has been completely destabilized, Iran has been strengthened and empowered, and the neo-conservative objective of democratic governments flourishing throughout the region remains as much of a pipedream as it was before.

George W. Bush's invasion of Iraq in 2003 was the greatest strategic military blunder in U.S. history, greater even than Vietnam. Iraq did not want or seek war with the United States. It had nothing to do with 9/11. America's crippling sanctions had destroyed their economy. Saddam had no weapons of mass destruction. The entire war was launched on lies and phony, half-baked evidence cherry-picked by Dick Cheney and his neo-con allies within the Bush Administration. And 5,000 Americans died, with more than 30,000 wounded. 200,000 Iraqi civilians also perished.

President Trump is right to want to put an end to this outrageous sacrifice of America's finest young men and women and the untold agony inflicted on their families, as well as those of innocent civilians. And, with America's debt clock nearing $23 trillion, we cannot afford these "wars of choice" any longer. It is time for America to end the silly Wilsonian crusades for world democracy, regime change, or whatever other high-sounding cliché the neo-cons conjure up. America's wars should be fought only as a last resort and only in defense of our borders or if there is a compelling and critical national interest truly at stake.

THE TAXPAYER RIP-OFF
CALLED "FOREIGN AID"

November 13, 2019

O F ALL THE WONDERFUL RATHOLES THE FEDERAL government has devised for tossing down billions of taxpayer dollars, none is more outrageous than so-called "foreign aid," an annual rip-off costing Americans more than $50 billion. And, that $50 billion does not include the hundreds of billions within the defense budget that are simply disguised foreign aid, especially to the NATO nations whose militaries we've been subsidizing for sixty years.

It is ironic that the Democrats' impeachment fantasy focused on this particular issue in regard to the nation of Ukraine and President Trump's apparent desire to link anti-corruption investigations to handing over our money to Kiev. Leave it to the Democrats to think they could inspire a national uprising against the President over what is undoubtedly the least popular federal spending program ever conceived. After all, how many of you approve of sending tens of billions of dollars abroad to nations and governments that you never heard of while our veterans are dying in the streets and we have record numbers of homeless people in our major cities?

You can search the U.S. Constitution high and low and find not one word authorizing the automatic annual transfer of taxpayer money to other countries. There is not and never has been any constitutional basis for foreign aid whatsoever.

Yet, ever since the end of World War II, we have spent more than $1.2 trillion on foreign aid. That monstrous figure represents the entire size of the federal budget during Ronald Reagan's second term.

A United Nations report produced in the mid-1990s analyzed the results of U.S. foreign aid spending in seventy countries. It found that every one of these countries was actually worse off than it was in 1980, most worse off in fact than in 1970. Clearly, sending American tax dollars to corrupt governments overseas does nothing to lift standards of living, unshackle command economies, or deliver freedom and prosperity to their people. In most cases, these funds just subsidize and maintain corrupt and socialist governments in power, throwing them a temporary lifeline that helps them avoid making the necessary structural changes in their economies, like establishing property rights and a free market pricing system. Give a man a fish, as opposed to teaching a man to fish....

A September 2002 White House report confirmed this, declaring that foreign aid "has often served to prop up failed policies, relieving the pressure for reform and perpetuating misery."

Let's look at a few more examples:

A 2003 report from a leading university in Bangladesh estimated that 75 percent of all foreign aid to that country is lost to corruption.

Northwestern University political economist Jeffrey Winters claims more than 50 percent of World Bank aid is lost to corruption in some African nations. Then-President Obasanjo of Nigeria said in 2002 that African leaders had stolen at least $140 billion from their people in the decades since independence.

A 2002 American Economic Review analysis concluded that "increases in foreign aid are associated with contemporaneous increases in corruption," and that "corruption is positively correlated with aid received from the United States."

And let's look at the mess in Afghanistan where we have been at war for twenty-plus years. According to the Defense Department's inspector general, more than $113 billion has been spent on nation-building in that land. Adjusted for inflation, that's $10 billion more than was spent to rebuild post-War Europe under the Marshall Plan! Most of that money was lost to waste, fraud, and abuse. The people of Afghanistan never even used one-third of the completed reconstruction projects and many of the other projects are in the hands of the Taliban. Sixteen of the twenty-one projects analyzed were judged to have deficiencies so severe that it was a danger for anyone to occupy them. The reports also cite unqualified contractor personnel, inferior materials, poor workmanship, and inadequate oversight. Even more appalling are news reports that former Afghan President Hamid Karzai would receive sacks full of CIA "ghost money" regularly in his office.

Yes, taxpayers, that's what you got for $113 billion!

Then we became engaged in a Democrat and Deep State-driven "constitutional crisis" over President Trump's apparent demands to attach a few strings to the transfer of American taxpayer money to the corrupt government of Ukraine. He actually asked that they fight corruption! Isn't that a novel idea? It certainly constitutes an impeachable offense. Adam Schiff, Nancy Pelosi and their ilk clearly believed your money should be distributed around the world to governments of their choosing, with no questions asked.

If fighting corruption and demanding accountability for the use of taxpayer money abroad constitutes a "quid pro quo," then count me in favor of the "quid pro quo," and while we're at it, count me in favor of terminating the unconstitutional foreign aid program altogether and returning those funds to the taxpayers from whom those funds were illegitimately confiscated.

THE CHINA SYNDROME

March 12, 2020

W HEN AIR FORCE ONE LANDED IN BEIJING IN February 1972, how many Americans could have envisioned that Richard Nixon's icebreaking trip to one of this nation's most ruthless enemies would eventually result in that enemy nation virtually seizing control of the world economy a half-century later?

At the time Nixon normalized relations with Communist China in 1972, Beijing was a virtual fourth-world economy, a great nation whose rich history and great potential was destroyed by the jackboot of totalitarianism. In twenty years, Mao had destroyed the country's economy, slaughtered 60 million innocents, brought his countrymen to the brink of nuclear war in Korea and unleashed the brutal upheaval of the Cultural Revolution. In comparison, the Republic of China on Taiwan had flourished since the end of the Chinese Civil War in 1949, a free and prosperous nation with one of Asia's strongest economies.

Nixon's opening to China was a Metternich-type act of international diplomacy intended to capitalize on the growing split between the Soviet Union and its former Asian client-state, as well as an effort to end the Vietnam War. Seven years later, President

Carter, in a monumental act of betrayal toward our old and loyal allies on Taiwan, carried Nixon's action to the next step and formally switched U.S. diplomatic recognition from Taipei to the Butchers of Beijing.

A new class of leaders had emerged in Communist China after the death of Mao in 1976, less wedded to doctrinaire Marxist-Leninist ideology and more committed to economic and military power. Leaders such as Deng Xiaoping saw the opportunities for attracting Western capital and investment to a nation impoverished and decimated from thirty years of Mao's rule. American capitalists were only too happy to cooperate, seeing the massive potential in a consumer market of 1 billion people still consigned to riding bicycles as their chief means of transportation. As Lenin once said, the Western capitalists would sell the Communists the rope with which the latter would hang them. Rope-selling began in earnest in the 1980s.

In 1985, the U.S. trade deficit with China was a paltry $6 million. Within four years, it had risen to $6 billion, and by 1999 it had skyrocketed to $68 billion. Throughout the 1980s and 1990s, under both Republican and Democrat administrations, Beijing was granted so-called "Most Favored Nation" trade status which provided for lower tariffs and other trade concessions, despite its sales of sensitive military technology to hostile actors and its continued human rights abuses, including the 1989 crackdown in Tiananmen Square, as well as its persecution of Christians. President Bill Clinton granted Communist China permanent MFN status in 2000 and helped usher in its entry into the World Trade Organization in 2001. After those actions, China's efforts to gain global economic supremacy moved into high gear with the clear and unqualified support of a United States government beholden to those giant corporations whose profits would soar as a result of off-sourcing their labor costs to a nation that still employed slave labor in many of its factories. Far from "free trade," the MFN-WTO policies of the Clinton, Bush, and Obama administrations involved the calculated and systematic stripping of America's manufacturing sector and shipping it to an enemy nation.

One by one, leading American industries from coal, steel and textiles to automobiles and electronics moved to China. China became the world's number one producer of steel, coal, and cars. In 2010, China's production of steel was nearly ten times that of the United States. Sixty thousand American factories were lost and 3.7 million jobs between 2001 and 2017. The trade deficit reached an all-time high of $420 billion in 2018 while the Economic Policy Institute reports that the wages of all non-college graduates dropped by $180 billion per year due to the China Syndrome.

And these job losses weren't simply based in the industrial heartland of Ohio, Michigan, and Pennsylvania, where boarded-up factories and ghost towns dominate the landscape and the opioid crisis overwhelms communities where hope was lost just as the jobs were lost: 1.2 million jobs vanished in the high-tech economy where Apple, IBM, HP and others saw unlimited profits in paying Chinese workers a fraction of the pay of their American cohorts, with 562,000 jobs lost in California alone.

The World Trade Organization – which is itself an unconstitutional entity as it cedes congressional control over international commerce to an unelected body of UN bureaucrats – was sold to Americans as a way of "keeping China in line."

It has done nothing of the sort. Beijing routinely flouts international trade standards as a matter of policy, from levying tariffs and non-tariff trade barriers to massive subsidies to state industries, lax labor and environmental law enforcement, currency manipulation, and outright theft of intellectual property. U.S. companies are often forced to hand over their trade secrets to do business on the mainland.

Communist China has a long-term plan to become the globe's number one economic superpower. It is called Project 2035. With a compliant, controlled, and cheap work force of 1.4 billion people, it can easily reach that objective unless it is forcefully confronted. The fact that a series of American politicians and policymakers of both parties have, for more than two decades, actively abetted and advanced Beijing's plans is little more than economic treason.

Not only have the livelihoods of millions of innocent working Americans been cruelly sacrificed to the gods of uber-profits, but our own financial and national security has been gravely endangered. Beijing has been America's banker for years, currently owning more than $1 trillion of our debt. If they stop buying our bonds, the dollar could crash. We are dependent on China for twenty of twenty-three strategic minerals, including rare earth minerals used for military equipment such as jet engines, lasers, satellites, and missile guidance systems. And, in the midst of the over-hyped COVID-19 crisis, we are dependent on China for hundreds of life-saving medications, including 97 percent of antibiotics.

It is way past time to end our dependence on Communist China. It is way past time to bring our supply chains back home. It is way past time to end the economic surrender to Beijing. Corporate America and the Communist Chinese regime are hooked at the hip. They would like nothing better than to bring down President Trump for threatening their unholy alliance. Don't think that the Coronavirus scare isn't part of their plan. If they can get Trump out of the way, they can return to business as usual and hand the keys of the global economy over to Xi Jinping. Let's not let them get away with it.

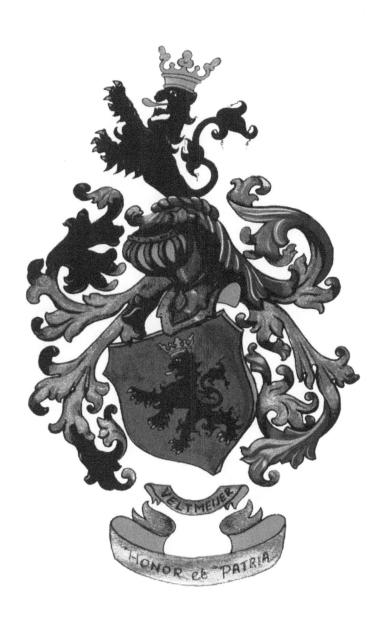

IMMIGRATION:

IMMIGRATION REFORM THAT WORKS

January 23, 2019

THE LAST TIME THE UNITED STATES HAD A FUNDA-
mental revision to our immigration laws was in 1965, when
Sen. Ted Kennedy decided it was time to consign our existing
immigration laws (enacted forty years earlier) to the ash heap
of history.

The Kennedy legislation replaced national origin quotas that
focused on attracting skilled immigrants from Europe to a much
more diverse policy that emphasized family unification (i.e.,
"chain migration") instead of skills. It also shifted the demographic
formula from the Old World to the Third World.

In 1986, the results of the Kennedy immigration law had created such a flood of *illegal* immigration that President Reagan
was persuaded to grant a massive amnesty to 5 million illegal
immigrants. At the time, Reagan believed he would get real
border security in exchange for the amnesty. He was misled, it
never happened.

Since 1986, the number of illegal immigrants in the country
has increased more than four-fold to over 22 million, possibly
as high as 30 million (10 percent of the U.S. population) costing
taxpayers $135 billion per year, more than what was spent to run

the entire federal government when John F. Kennedy was in the White House. These are just the "hard" costs, in terms of federal, state and local health, education and welfare spending. It does not include the incalculable costs of lost lives and shattered families due to drugs smuggled into the country or to homicides and rapes committed by illegal aliens. If this is not a crisis, what is?

The politicians in Washington have failed time after time over the last several decades to address this crisis. Multiple attempts at so-called "comprehensive immigration reform" have crashed and burned.

Most of these past efforts have failed because of the special interests and political agendas involved. Democrats have demanded additional amnesties and paths to "legalization" that would ensure ample numbers of new Democratic Party voters. Grassroots Republicans have insisted on ironclad border security and rejected amnesty for lawbreakers. Corporate Republicans eager for cheap labor have tended to side with the Democrats in wanting to take a softer approach to the issue.

We now face a bare knuckles battle over President Trump's Border Wall, a weeks-long government shutdown, and thousands of migrants marching in caravans to invade our country's southern border. Could there be a better time or a more ideal opportunity to declare a "time out" on the war of words and political posturing and consider real immigration reform that is just plain common sense?

There are three critical components of sound immigration reform that prioritizes the interests of the American people.

The first and foremost is obviously border security. The security of our southern border must be ensured before moving on to the second component, the status of the 22 million illegal immigrants living in the U.S. The third component is who we want in our country and why.

Who are the best people to determine what is needed to secure the border? Chuck Schumer? Nancy Pelosi? President Trump? Certainly, the men and women on the front lines are the best positioned to make this determination: the Border Patrol. We should let the Border Patrol decide the best course to seal the border to crime, gangs, and drugs. If that means a wall or physical barrier in those areas where topography and terrain permit, then it should be built. If it means drones, sensors, and other new technologies, so be it. If it means more boots on the ground, let's give the Border Patrol what it needs. If it requires using assets of the U.S. military, let's do it. Let's give the folks who face this crisis each and every day the opportunity to craft a master plan for border security and fund that plan in full.

After the border is secured to the greatest extent possible (recognizing that no plan would be 100 percent effective) and *only* after should we move on to discussing the status of the 22 million-plus illegal immigrants already in the country. Here is a possible solution:

The 22 million illegal immigrants can be given six months to register in a national registry to apply for jobs that employers need filled but where there is a shortage of American workers because of the booming economy, low unemployment, etc. This would prevent the competition for jobs and wage suppression among low and unskilled American workers that unrestricted immigration normally causes. If they do not register within six months or there are no jobs for them, they must voluntarily return to their home country within one year or be deported. They would **not** be eligible for any taxpayer-paid benefits during that one-year period.

In similar fashion, employers would be required to sign in to a national job registry indicating the jobs they need filled and the reasons they cannot find enough American workers to fill them. This registry would be matched to the first one, creating a database of foreign workers to fill the U.S. jobs that cannot be staffed by sufficient numbers of qualified American workers.

After five years of working in the U.S. in jobs where there is a *verified* shortage of American workers, paying taxes, and having a clean criminal record, the illegal immigrants can apply to be legal residents (not citizens) via green card.

After obtaining green cards (paying taxes, maintaining a clean criminal record, learning English, etc.), they may eventually apply for citizenship, but they must go to the back of the line and apply through the normal process behind everyone else who has already applied legally and is awaiting acceptance of their applications.

Such an approach would accomplish what America really needs right now: immigrants to fill jobs that genuinely need to be filled by employers (as in the agriculture industry), not immigrants taking the jobs of American citizens or legal immigrants or exerting downward pressure on wages. If such a job to immigrant match cannot be made and verified as genuine, the illegal alien must return to his nation of origin.

Under this plan, there would be no amnesties of any kind. No "paths" to citizenship, other than a *possible* opportunity to eventually apply in the normal manner as legal immigrants are mandated to do.

The third component has to address legal immigration and define who we, as a sovereign nation, want in our country and why. Every year, the United States accepts more than 1 million legal immigrants to our shores. We must come to a consensus as a country whether this number is too high, whether it discourages rapid assimilation, and whether it unfairly victimizes American workers. We should consider significantly reducing levels of legal immigration to permit faster assimilation, restrict such immigration to skilled workers who will contribute to our economy (rather than simply seek government assistance) and *only* where a genuine shortage of labor actually warrants it.

Obviously, there are other issues related to immigration that must be discussed, such as "birth tourism" under the Fourteenth Amendment (something that would have shocked and stunned the authors of that Amendment), the atrocity of "sanctuary cities" that shield hardened criminals and gang leaders from the law and victimize innocent populations, *both* native and immigrant, and the welfare state magnets that draw foreign nationals to our borders. Many of these issues are constitutional in origin, would ignite long drawn-out battles in the federal courts, or require a total reexamination of the role of the federal government in health, education, and welfare since the 1960s. They need to be addressed at some point, but it won't happen quickly or painlessly.

My proposals offer some basic, but essential, common-sense solutions that the American people and their representatives in Congress can and should rally around, for the sake of national security and personal safety for our citizens and economic security for our American workers and their families.

IMMIGRATION AND THE NATION-STATE

June 14, 2019

A S THE CRISIS ON AMERICA'S SOUTHERN BORDER intensifies and worsens, it is highly appropriate to revisit the issue of immigration, both legal and illegal. This is a controversial topic and the socialist Democratic Party and its megaphones in the mainstream media wish to silence any rational discussion of this subject with a single pejorative: "racist." Yet, immigration is an issue that is inevitably linked to the greater issues of national sovereignty and national identity. It is really a matter of the survival of the nation-state itself.

On the eve of Patrick Buchanan's challenge to President Bush in the 1992 Republican primaries, he did an interview on David Brinkley's Sunday program on ABC. He asked an interesting question. What if tomorrow, Virginia was suddenly flooded with a million Englishmen or a million Zulus from Africa. Which group would be easier to assimilate and create fewer problems for the people of Virginia? Of course, the left predictably said this was a racist query. But was it really? Or was it a reasonable question?

The simple answer to Buchanan's question, one that almost any person would offer, is that it would be easier for Virginia to assimilate a million Englishmen. After all, the United States of America were originally thirteen colonies of England. The colonists were ruled by the English king. They spoke the English language and followed English common law. The first settlers to America came from England. Yes, the Pilgrims were indeed from England, not El Salvador!

Of course, to the open borders crowd, the mere suggestion that some people might be easier to assimilate than others is indicative of a "racist" mentality. Globalists — like the billionaire elitist, Nazi collaborator and currency manipulator, George Soros — who reject the very idea of the nation-state and national sovereignty envision a borderless world with uncontrolled mass migration of peoples and cultures. After all, in what pathetically passes as the mind of the Left, that is their "right." Nations are just artificial constructs; they are as easily erased as created. A person in Uganda or Sri Lanka has just as much right to be a citizen of Germany or France as an individual born and raised in those countries. The European Union itself is a ham-handed attempt to abolish the nation-state and it has resulted in the once-Christian nations of Europe being overwhelmed by Muslim migrants from North Africa. With increasing speed, the nations of the Old World are seeing their national identities and cultures subordinated to the European superstate. Churches are replaced by mosques. Mohammed becomes the most popular name for newborn boys in Great Britain. A Tower of Babel of languages overtakes London, Paris, and Rome. Cardinal Robert Sarah – an African – warns that the West will soon disappear and Islam will reign in the nations that produced Shakespeare, Dante, Michelangelo, Chopin and Vincent Van Gogh.

Now, what if the shoe were on the other foot? What if tens of millions of Britons, French, Germans, and Italians invaded the Islamic nations of the Middle East? What if these European nationals engaged in a recolonization of the lands they largely abandoned after World War II: Libya, Algeria, Morocco, Iraq, Tunisia, Egypt. Would the inhabitants of those lands welcome their former conquerors back, to tear down their mosques and shrines and replace them with Catholic cathedrals and Protestant churches? Would they welcome them back to impose their European languages and Christian holidays? Would they applaud having their systems of law and government dismantled and replaced with Western representative democracies? Our former nation-building President George W. Bush tried to do something along those lines a decade ago in Iraq and it didn't turn out too well.

It seems as if it is perfectly acceptable to abolish the language, religion, culture, and history of the West, but it would be an appalling violation of the rights and self-determination of the Muslim peoples of the Middle East to impose Western values and systems upon them. Sounds like a double standard to me.

We face the same situation in America with the problem of illegal immigration and the convoys of migrant caravans that continue to invade our nation. The Democrats in Congress refuse to change the crazy asylum laws that are permitting this invasion. They refuse to give the President the resources to secure the border. Some of them even call for tearing down existing barriers and deep-sixing ICE.

Why? Are they not Americans too? The unfortunate answer is that they too are globalists. They don't believe in the nation-state. That means they reject America as a unique Constitutional Republic based on the systems of language, government and law we inherited from our British ancestors. No, to them, America is merely a slab of land separated by two oceans. It is a land born of white male privilege, slavery, inequality, and colonialism. Those who achieved financial or economic success here did it, not because of skill or sweat, but because they stole the wealth of someone else. Therefore, why is America worth fighting for? Why defend its borders? Let everyone in and let them bring their poverty, crime, gangs, and foreign languages and traditions with them. There is no need to assimilate them. We will just let the American taxpayers pay for education in their native tongue and their health care, while ensuring they have access to welfare, food stamps, and subsidized housing. We will guarantee that road signs and ballots will be written in Spanish and that they have driver's licenses. We will let greedy employers hire them over native-born Americans without penalty. They will have all the perks and privileges of citizenship by simply crossing the border. After all, what is American citizenship if we are all "citizens of the world"? Let's just turn the United States into the "polyglot boardinghouse for the world" that President Theodore Roosevelt condemned more than a century ago.

Of course, we go back to the double-standard. If Catholic Mexico were tomorrow flooded by tens of millions of blond, blue-eyed Protestant Scandinavians, would Mexico still be Mexico? Would the Mexican government permit its religion, language, culture, and history to be abolished in favor of a new cultural paradigm imposed by Swedes, Norwegians, and Danes? Would the Mexican government rewrite its laws to accommodate the newly arrived immigrants? Would they be taught in Mexican schools the language of Eric the Red and the history of the Vikings? Would aebelskiver take the place of flan? Would they receive "free" public services?

There is nothing "racist" about respecting the unique, God-given differences among the many peoples of the world. That *is* the diversity that the liberals are always shouting about. There is nothing "racist" about believing in the nation-state and the preservation of national identity. Religion, language, culture, and history define who we are, where we came from, and what we believe.

They are what we see in the faces of our children and grandchildren and in the photographs of our parents and grandparents. We have a right and obligation to protect and defend our heritage from the globalist destroyers who are the true racists – the would-be world controllers who would abolish all races, religions, and cultures to create their godless New World Order.

IT'S TIME TO TERMINATE THE H1-B VISA PROGRAM

April 29, 2020

Resident Trump's recent decision to suspend legal immigration into the United States as a result of the COVID-19 crisis should be applauded as a first step toward addressing America's out-of-control legal immigration system. However, does the President's action go far enough? Does it do enough to protect American workers and American jobs at a time when the virus has tanked the economy and sent over 26 million Americans into unemployment lines?

For years now, the United States has taken in more *legal* immigrants each year than every other nation in the world combined. That's more than 1 million annually. What has been the impact of such a high level of immigration, unprecedented since the wave of Irish, Italian, German and Jewish immigrants flooded our shores in the late 19th and early 20th centuries?

First of all, we know wages in this country have been virtually stagnant since 1998 and have only started to rise slightly since President Trump took office. We know that is indisputable that high levels of immigration suppress wages. Libertarian theorists may like to challenge this fact, but it is true. It is simply a matter of basic economics. When the supply of something rises, its price falls and vice versa. When the supply of labor rises, its price – meaning wages — drops. It is no coincidence that wages and living standards for working Americans increased dramatically – except for the period of the Great Depression – when immigration levels were essentially frozen between 1924 and 1965. Employers had to pay more because the labor supply was tight.

Unfortunately, the final version of the President's proclamation did not address the issue of temporary foreign workers in the United States and the notorious H1-B Visa program. It is believed the original version sought to suspend these temporary visas as well, but that aggressive lobbying by the cheap labor lobby of Corporate America succeeded in having it omitted in the final decree. This is a gaping omission.

The H1-B Visa program is an enemy of working and middle-class Americans. It is the program through which hundreds of thousands of foreign workers from India, Communist China, Vietnam and other nations are imported into the United States to take jobs in high-tech, health care, and other industries that should go to American workers. Every year more than 100,000 such foreign workers are brought here and allowed to stay for up to six years. It is estimated that there are at least 650,000 such workers in this country at any given time. And, in 2018 alone, U.S. businesses and corporations tried to outsource as many as 420,000 jobs through the program. Between 2007 and 2017, it is estimated that 2.7 million Americans lost their jobs to so-called "temporary" foreign workers.

According to Joe Guzzardi of Progressives for Immigration Reform:

The H1-B scam has gone on long enough. Over the last three decades, the H1-B has displaced tens of thousands of experienced U.S. tech workers and has created financial and emotional heartache for Americans who have lost their jobs to younger, less-skilled but cheaper-to-employ workers.

Guzzardi cites several prominent Silicon Valley companies who "phase out" older employees for younger, cheaper workers from abroad, including Apple, Facebook, Google, HP, LinkedIn, and Tesla. Ron Hira of the Economic Policy Institute has written that the H1B Visa program and its L-1 cousin contain loopholes that "have made it too easy to bring in cheaper foreign workers, with ordinary skills, who directly substitute for, rather than complement, workers already in the country. They are clearly displacing and denying opportunities to U.S. workers." In 2019, we learned of AT&T's plans to lay off thousands of workers while making them train their foreign replacements. Many of these workers have been with the company for more than a decade and won't be offered severance or early retirement.

India has greatly benefited from the H-1B Visa program, at the expense of the United States. By rolling out the red carpet to Indian engineering students who then take the jobs of American IT workers and later return to India, we have enabled a massive high-tech boom in India. Displaced Americans are forced to take jobs in non-computer science careers, thus weakening our own home-grown high-tech industry. Exports of IT goods from the U.S. has declined steadily since 1995 while India has enjoyed a spectacular surge.

Congressman Paul Gosar of Arizona has written to the President, asking him to suspend all the temporary foreign worker Visa programs while we work ourselves through the current pandemic-induced economic cataclysm. He is right. Additionally, I would argue that even in a period of unparalleled prosperity, such schemes should not be permitted to displace American workers or used as a means by which corporations suppress wage levels. As I argued in one of my earliest OpEds, immigrant labor should be brought into the United States only under the strictest conditions, specifically verification that the jobs to be filled cannot under any circumstance be filled by the existing U.S. labor force and not as a way to hold down wages. Only where a genuine shortage of labor or where a perishable commodity exists, as in the agricultural economy, for example, can these programs be justified.

President Trump's Executive Order may be updated in sixty days. We should urge him to turn a deaf ear to the selfish appeals of the Business Roundtable and the Chamber of Commerce and instead listen to the cries of American fathers and mothers being crushed by the current shutdown. It's time to terminate the H1-B program and its noxious cousins in their current form and time to put American workers first.

THE HEALTH CARE COSTS OF OPEN BORDERS

February 19, 2019

A S A PHYSICIAN, I AM CONCERNED ABOUT THE HEALTH and well-being of my patients.

I am similarly concerned about the escalating costs of health care that are burdening middle- and working-class Americans. Each and every day, I see financially hard-pressed or uninsured Americans – many of them veterans – who cannot afford to be treated and are not eligible for government assistance. I can cite a few examples of our first responders and veterans who were forced to hold fundraisers to come up with the money to pay their medical bills or that I had to turn back to the streets because there was "no room at the inn" for them.

The irony of this situation is that while American citizens are being denied appropriate care, illegal immigrants are often receiving top-dollar care, courtesy of the U.S. taxpayers.

The Federation for American Immigration Reform (FAIR) estimates that it costs the federal government more than $17 billion to care for the medical needs of those individuals who are unlawfully residing in our country. This figure includes the costs of uncompensated hospital expenditures, Medicaid births,

Medicaid fraud, and Medicaid for U.S.-born children of illegal immigrants (so-called "anchor babies"). State costs are pegged at more than $12 billion.

Technically, federal law is supposed to prohibit the expenditure of money to pay for the medical care of illegal aliens. However, numerous loopholes in the laws (especially Emergency Medicaid) mean taxpayers foot the bills anyway. Far-left "progressive" Democrats like California Gov. Gavin Newsom and New York City Mayor Bill De Blasio now demand taxpayers pay for the cradle to grave medical care of all undocumented immigrants.

This is wrong because it means that individuals who have no right to be in the United States are often being prioritized over American citizens. Let me cite a few examples from my work as a physician as well as from my colleagues:

A Mexican national in his thirties approached the border and asked a Border Patrol agent if he could call 911 because he was sick. He wound up at a San Diego hospital where he was diagnosed with necrotizing pancreatitis related to alcoholism, spent almost three months in ICU and walked away having incurred costs of over $1 million, which will be absorbed by the hospital or charged to U.S. taxpayers.

Four days after suffering a stroke in Mexico, a Mexican national was brought to a local hospital. He spent six weeks there and later was released to a Board and Care facility with speech therapy, physical therapy, occupational therapy, the works – courtesy of U.S. taxpayers, despite the fact that this individual had previously been found by immigration authorities to have committed MediCal fraud.

An Iraqi man was brought to a local hospital directly from the San Diego International Airport. He needed emergency cardiac bypass surgery. He received it at a cost of over $350,000. No bill. No collection agency. No bankruptcy.

While non-citizens are receiving top-end care at our American medical facilities and simply walking away from huge bills the hospital has to either write off or the taxpayers wind up on the hook for, hard-working Americans are being denied care because they lack health insurance or the right kind of health insurance. Many veterans find themselves in this position and I see it on a regular basis. There was recently a situation where a patriotic first responder was forced to have his fire department colleagues host a fundraiser for him so he could pay the deductible necessary for him to undergo life-saving pancreatic surgery. Similarly, a young homeless American veteran who required partial amputation of his foot due to uncontrolled diabetes was refused placement to a skilled nursing facility because he lacked insurance – being discharged back to the streets!

In addition, a real potential public health emergency looms large due to once-eradicated diseases being brought into the United States by unscreened illegal immigrants. In recent years, we have seen a surge in cases of malaria, dengue, leprosy, Chagas disease, scabies, flesh-eating bacteria, and tuberculosis. We are also witnessing diseases little-seen outside the Third World, like schistosomiasis, Guinea Worm infection, cysticercosis, and Morgellon's. According to the Centers for Disease Control (CDC):

Studies have identified the importance of cross-border movement in the transmission of various diseases, including HIV, measles, pertussis, rubella, rabies, Hepatitis A, influenza, tuberculosis, shigellosis, syphilis, Mycobacterium bovis infection, brucellosis, and foodborne diseases, such as infections associated with raw cheese and produce. ("The Migrant Caravan of Diseases," *American Thinker,* November 28, 2018)

It should be noted that the CDC does *not* recommend across-the-board screening for everyone entering the United States, nor does CDC test for latent tuberculosis (LTBI). In Indiana, almost one-quarter of the nearly 2,000 refugees admitted to the state in 2015 did *not* complete post-annual medical screenings.

The Association of American Physicians and Surgeons has weighed in on the topic:

> What invisible travelers are accompanying them? And what infections are already here in the millions of illegals already dispersed throughout the country? In the past, waves of immigrants from Europe were stopped at Ellis Island, medically examined, and quarantined long enough to be sure they were not incubating a contagious disease. Procedures are less rigorous today, and, of course, those who enter illegally are not screened at all. ("The Migrant Caravan of Diseases," *American Thinker,* November 28, 2018)

In recent months, the medical profession has been stumped by a polio-like disease that is striking down mostly young children around the country. It is called acute flaccid myelitis (AFM) and is believed to be caused by a virus. This flu-like illness progresses to difficulty in swallowing, slurred speech, and sudden limb weakness. While polio itself has been wiped out in most parts of the world, it is still endemic in Pakistan, Afghanistan, and Nigeria. It has also re-emerged in Venezuela. There is a high likelihood that AFM is being spread by the migrant caravans invading our country. We already know from news reports that many of the migrants (especially the children) are sick from a variety of illnesses. Most are not vaccinated and come from countries where public health and sanitary standards are low.

The question arises: Why would any responsible government expose its people to these diseases? Perhaps it is because our "open borders" ruling class is largely isolated from such problems, as they and their children are tucked away in their "white-privilege" neighborhoods and exclusive private schools where the biggest challenge might be which country club to choose for a "sweet sixteen" party.

As a physician and as a parent, I reject the political agenda of America's liberal elites who would endanger the health of our fellow citizens and elevate the health care needs of illegal immigrants over our veterans and other native-born Americans and legal immigrants. In their relentless quest for political power and votes from the illegal immigrant population, these elites are willing to let your families suffer and even die from imported diseases and maladies or the lack of affordable health care which is readily provided to those who have broken into our country. It is outrageous and represents the most twisted set of priorities imaginable. As a doctor, I'm in the business of healing people and saving lives; I should not have to deal with the political power plays of the Democratic Party and its shameful leadership at the emergency room door.

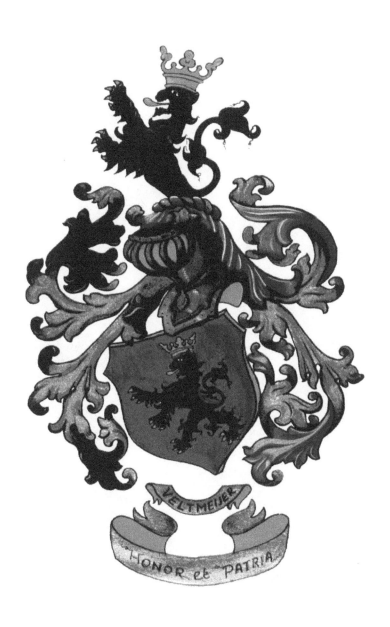

VELTMEIJER

HONOR et PATRIA

DEMOCRATIC PARTY

DEMOCRATIC PARTY ELITES ARE THE MODERN SLAVE MASTERS

January 2, 2019

A S A CHILD IMMIGRANT FROM SOUTH AMERICA, I can only watch with anguish as the migrant caravans from Guatemala, Honduras, and El Salvador march through Mexico and seek to enter the United States.

However, my anguish is not because I believe the U.S. government is in error by strictly enforcing our nation's laws and blocking a foreign legion from violating our sovereignty. The Trump Administration is absolutely correct that illegal entry into the United States must be stopped; if the migrants have a legitimate claim for asylum due to political or religious persecution, they have to apply at a valid port of entry and be processed legally. I should know. I came to America legally, waiting years to get a visa. If there needs to be some reform of the immigration system, it is not by erasing national borders and national sovereignty.

Every country has an inherent right to determine who it accepts into its bosom. This is fundamental to the very concept of nationhood. Most of the migrants are economic refugees and the U.S. obviously cannot absorb every person on the planet who thinks they can get a better job here.

Yet, the existence of a welfare state in the United States since Lyndon Johnson's "Great Society" of the mid-1960s has done exactly what Nobel Prize-winning economist Milton Friedman once argued was impossible: "open borders with a welfare state." It is impossible and unsustainable because such a system will automatically attract most of the world's population to our shores to gain access to the liberal social benefits we offer, from free education and health care to food stamps, welfare, and even subsidies to attend college. Now, San Francisco even maintains that the right to vote should follow.

Having come to the United States from Ecuador, I know a little about how socialist welfare states destroy societies. Look at Venezuela as a prime example. An oil-rich nation, once the pride of the continent, is now an economic basket case that can't print additional zeros fast enough on its worthless currency. This is the result of socialism.

Socialism does not uplift individuals; it impoverishes them. It does not raise living standards; it decimates them. It does not advance human potential, but, as Franklin D. Roosevelt said, it subtly destroys the human spirit. This failed ideology—of whatever variety— has never worked successfully anywhere and never will. Neither Bernie Sanders' $30 trillion "Medicare for all" nor the latest giveaway scheme mouthed by Alexandria Ocasio-Cortez can succeed because as Margaret Thatcher noted, "You eventually run out of other people's money." Or, the ink on the printing presses runs dry.

Of course, socialism itself has never been a system intended to help anyone, other than the elite ruling class of a nation who sees it not as a way to raise up the poor and working class, but as a way to keep them down and under control, stifling their ambition and upward mobility. Socialism is slavery or serfdom, pure and simple. I'm from South America, so I know a little about tyranny.

And socialism is tyranny. Even Marx saw socialism as only the phase preceding communism. However, far from the "withering away of the state," socialism's final stage –communism — only leads to a totalitarian terror state that bulldozes human liberty and enslaves the human soul.

The socialism (or what is currently mislabeled "progressivism") that the Democratic Party offers new arrivals from abroad – be they legal immigrants or illegal aliens – is not the freedom they crave, but the slave state of political and economic regimentation lorded over by a ruling elite that seeks only to expand and maintain its power. That is exactly what the Pelosis, Schumers and company seek: not to help a suffering population or rescue those escaping poverty or persecution abroad, but to use these unfortunate people in a cynical political power play to solidify their electoral position through creating a permanently dependent underclass willing to trade its votes for the promise of cradle to grave security. It is an illusion and it is despicable. Yet, it is the history of the Democratic Party in America for more than a century, from being the party of Southern slaveholders to being the party of Tammany Hall, which cruelly manipulated our earlier generations of immigrants, exchanging jobs for votes. They are still at it, now exchanging food stamps and Medicaid for votes.

The Democratic Party detests the idea of its immigrant underclass becoming self-reliant and independent, business owners and entrepreneurs. That may lead them to becoming Republicans, after all!

Far from being the party of the working people, the Democratic Party today is the party of the billionaire plutocrat elites – the Steyers and Soroses and Bloombergs – which draws its greatest strength from the millionaire enclaves of Silicon Valley, Manhattan, and suburban Washington. D.C. And these are the folks whose aspirations for the migrant caravans yearning for the American

Dream is to consign them to a future of despair and dependency where their hopes for the future remain buried in sub-minimum wage jobs and tending to the lawns, toilets, and estates of their present-day slave masters.

HAS THE DEMOCRATIC PARTY GONE CRAZY?

April 2, 2019

MILLIONS OF AMERICANS, INCLUDING COUNTLESS numbers of cradle Democrats from our nation's heart-land, are scratching their heads in wonder and disbelief at today's Democratic Party. Even considering that party's rather unsavory past in regards to slavery, Jim Crow, and the Ku Klux Klan, the present currents within the party of Jefferson and Jackson are downright looney.

For decades, the Democratic Party has heralded itself as the champion of working and middle-class wage-earners, while the Republican Party was pigeonholed as the party of big business and the wealthy. Yet, the most prominent representatives of the party now, personified by the likes of Bernie Sanders, Kamala Harris and media darling Queen Alexandria Ocasio-Big Mouth, would literally wipe out millions of middle-class jobs in America's most important industries to carry out their fight against so-called "cli-mate change." If anyone works in the oil and gas industry, the auto-mobile industry, or works for an airline or on an aircraft assembly line, you better prepare for the unemployment line if these New Democrats have their way. If you're a farmer, you better let your land lie idle, as Queen Alexandria is coming for your tractor. If you are one of 170 million Americans who receive your medical coverage through your employer, forget it. And, if you are one of the many thousands of Americans working in the health insurance field, clean out your desk. As a physician, my job would be nationalized and I would no longer work for my patients, but for the government.

The so-called "Green New Deal" that has been embraced by most of the Democratic presidential candidates and dozens of members of Congress demonstrates how truly radical and dangerous these New Democrats have become. With a price tag that is five times the size of the U.S. economy and would cost every American household $65,000 per year, this scheme would crash the American economy while building trains to Hawaii and putting government bureaucrats in charge of your Quarter Pounder consumption. It would unleash widespread poverty throughout our land. Is this what the party of Franklin D. Roosevelt and John F. Kennedy has come to? Unfortunately, this is not a joke; these people are deadly serious. They truly admire the vicious totalitarian socialist and communist states of the past and present.

Bernie Sanders honeymooned in the Soviet Union and praised bread lines. As an immigrant from Ecuador who actually stood in bread lines, I really think American supermarkets are far superior. Others have glorified Castro's Cuba and refuse to condemn Nicholas Maduro, the despot who is starving the people of Venezuela. To people like Bernie Sanders, Pocahontas, and Ocasio-Big Mouth, deprivation and suffering is really okay as long as *they* fly in private jets and own multiple homes, usually surrounded by gates. These Democrats have far more in common with Joseph Stalin, Mao Zedong, and Fidel Castro than they do with Roosevelt, Kennedy or even Lyndon Johnson.

FDR's New Deal, which the current crazies in the party have expropriated for their wacky plan, had many flaws but it certainly did not challenge the fundamental basis of the American economy: free market capitalism. Prior generations of Democrats sought not to abolish capitalism but take off some of its rough edges, to help the very people whose jobs the New Democrats now want to abolish. FDR did not want a "guaranteed income" for people unwilling to work. To the contrary, he believed welfare should be a temporary program only, otherwise he compared it to a narcotic that would destroy the human soul. Likewise, President Kennedy would be appalled to see the direction his party has taken. JFK was an advocate of economic growth and job creation through cutting tax rates, not raising them up to 90 percent or higher as proposed by some of the party's most addle-brained leaders.

Franklin D. Roosevelt forged the modern Democratic Party based on the tragedy of the Great Depression. It was a coalition, as all successful political movements generally are. It consisted of poor, rural Southern whites, African-Americans, union members, and Northern white Catholics and ethnics, like the Irish, Italians, and Poles. The Republican Party of that day was best described as the Episcopal Church at prayer. FDR's four successful presidential campaigns plus the Democrats' ability to hold Congress uninterruptedly for forty years was based on maintaining the support of this coalition of voters. While that coalition fractured slightly at the presidential level in the 1950s, due to the bipartisan appeal of the World War II hero, President Dwight D. Eisenhower, it did not start to crumble until the decisive election of 1968. 1968 – the year of America's collective nervous breakdown—saw working-class whites and union members defect in large numbers to Republican Richard Nixon and independent George Wallace. Combined, they captured 57 percent of the popular vote. The vote for Democrat Hubert Humphrey – LBJ's loyal vice president – was just 43 percent, eighteen points lower than Johnson's vote four years earlier, perhaps the peak of the party's electoral strength and public mandate. Yet, as a result of riots and civil unrest and the Vietnam War, that mandate collapsed in just forty-eight months. All the high hopes of LBJ's "Great Society" were buried in the jungles of Southeast Asia.

What happened? The "hard hats" and union members who were patriotic and culturally conservative were angered and outraged at what they saw as the outright anarchy that appeared to have gripped the nation: flags being burned, cities set aflame, and long-haired hippies and yippies running wild, preaching free love and the wonders of tripping on LSD. They left a Democratic Party that seemed to have lost control of the country and flocked to the law and order messages of Nixon and Wallace. Nixon, of course, was elected.

By 1972, the inmates had taken over the asylum of the party and it lurched far left, nominating triple A (Abortion, Acid and Amnesty) candidate George McGovern at a wild Miami convention where traditional Democrats were uninvited and Red China's murderous dictator, Mao, received votes for vice president. Sound familiar? The party's platform was so extreme that Big Labor, the historic heart and soul, not to mention checkbook of the party, walked away. As did millions of their members, earning Richard Nixon a forty-nine-state landslide re-election.

Is history repeating itself? Tens of millions of old-school Democrats whose forebears enlisted in FDR's New Deal army have permanently left the party. They are Catholics. They are Protestants. They are Irish. They are Italians. They are suburban. They are rural. What they aren't are socialists or communists. The party's dwindling support now relies almost exclusively on newly arrived Latino immigrants (the reason the party now supports completely "open borders," which also forces down the wages of the workers the Democrats claim to represent), African-Americans, and the Jewish community. And, only by importing millions more from south of the border does the party have any chance of empowering itself for generations.

However, the winds of radical socialism blow in many directions. President Trump's support among African-Americans reached new highs as unemployment fell to new lows. The President's approval rating among Hispanics has reached 40 percent. And Jewish voters who normally voted 70 percent to 80 percent for Democratic candidates may now be rethinking their allegiance to a party that winks and smiles at anti-Semitism.

If the Democratic Party nominates one of its radical extremists in 2020, offering voters a platform that prohibits cars and planes, wants to tax them at 90 percent, takes away their medical coverage, forces them on to all vegan diets, and legalizes infanticide, expect additional defections from what remains of the old "New Deal" coalition – including millions of African-Americans, Latinos and Jews – and a second term for Donald J. Trump.

DEMOCRATS: THE PARTY OF INFANTICIDE

April 11, 2019

MILLIONS OF AMERICAS WERE SICKENED AND appalled as the left-wing governor of New York signed legislation authorizing abortion up to the moment of birth. Governor Cuomo's fellow Democrats cheered lustily as his pen met paper. Similarly, the Democratic governor of Virginia, who claims to be a physician and who ridiculed African-Americans while in medical school, spoke casually of allowing an infant to die after delivery, as he endorsed legislation in his state which would have permitted abortion after birth. Not to be undone in their rush to embrace infanticide, all but three Democrats in the U.S. Senate voted to reject a bill that would have saved the lives of babies who survived abortions.

As a physician myself and as a father, I can only feel shame for my adopted country where such barbaric actions could take place and where one of our major political parties embraces abortion as a holy sacrament, the all-important ritual of what can only be called a death cult of human sacrifice. Today's Democrats would make even the Aztecs blush.

The sorry saga of abortion in the United States can be traced to the cultural nihilism of the late 1960s, which led a number of states to liberalize their laws against abortion. Let us recall that under President John F. Kennedy, abortion was a crime in all fifty states. California Governor Ronald Reagan agonized and agonized over signing the Beilenson Therapeutic Abortion Act in 1967. He finally signed it, very reluctantly and regretted it for the rest of his life. He never envisioned that it would be used to allow abortions for almost any reason a psychiatrist or other mental health "professional" could dream up. New York followed in 1970.

However, January 22, 1973, was the true day that should live in infamy for anyone who believes in the sanctity of innocent human life. On that day, seven justices on the U.S. Supreme Court – many of them senescent fossils from the Roosevelt and Eisenhower eras – usurped the role of fifty popularly elected state legislatures and imposed their vision of abortion law on the nation through an abomination called *Roe v. Wade*. Legislating from the bench, Justice Harry Blackmun constructed a complicated framework of trimesters (which he admitted were "arbitrary") to declare that the so-called "right to privacy" is "broad enough" to encompass a woman killing her unborn baby. It is interesting to note that the "right to privacy" does not actually exist. It is found nowhere in the United States Constitution. *Nowhere*. It's one of those things, as President Trump would say, that "they just make up." And, this invented "right" has cost the lives of 60 million unborn Americans over the last forty-five years, which is about equal to the entire population of Italy. Think of the contribution those 60 million souls would have made to our country and to the world, in terms of math, medicine, science and technology, theatre, the arts, and yes, even politics. Their contributions alone to the Social Security system might have made the program solvent.

For today's socialist Democrats, January 22, 1973 should be a national holiday, possibly as a replacement for Thanksgiving. However, even the *Roe v. Wade* decision is not anywhere sufficient to satisfy the radical extremists who now control the Democrat Party. *Roe* only permitted unrestricted abortion in the first trimester but accepted some state limitations in the second and third trimesters. Today's Democrats want abortion for any reason, at any time, up to the moment of birth and even *after* birth. This is indeed the insane agenda of a party that is completely off the rails.

Of course, the Democratic Party, which is largely funded by the abortion industry and Planned Parenthood (which sells the body parts of aborted babies in a particularly gruesome fundraiser) wants people to believe this is just a matter of women's rights. Of course, at least half of the 60 million abortions in this country terminated the lives of baby girls. Women themselves are largely victims of the very profitable abortion industry as they are lied to repeatedly to prevent them from understanding the true consequences of their actions and the dangers abortion poses to women's health, both physical and mental. As a physician, I can state categorically that abortion poses a greater risk to women than delivery, even if it is a complicated delivery or a deformed or disabled child is involved. With the technologies available today, an unborn baby can survive on its own at five months and there is almost never a threat to a mother's life by carrying a baby to term.

The socialist Democrats have come full circle, from a time when abortion was illegal and considered a horrendous crime under their party heroes, Franklin D. Roosevelt and John F. Kennedy, to today when they cheer Andrew Cuomo and Ralph Northam in signing or endorsing abortion to the moment of birth or after. In adopting their radical pro-abortion program, the socialist Democrats are just one step away from actually forcing abortions on women as they have done for years in Communist

China to enforce their draconian "one-child" policy. Especially if Alexandria Ocasio-Big Mouth decrees that future population growth (except through illegal immigration) be stopped, as it might contribute to "climate change."

After all, coercion is what socialism is all about. And Bernie Sanders, Kamala Harris, and Queen Alexandria are just contemporary examples of history's greatest despots who seek power and control over the rest of us who, once our firearms are confiscated, will be unable to resist.

THE THIRD DEMOCRAT PRESIDENTIAL DEBATE

July 9, 2019

Castro: All future presidential debates should be conducted in Spanish.

Beto: Si, si, senor

Warren: And we need a federal program to fund interpreters for the English-speaking

DeBlasio: English should no longer be taught in American schools. It is a colonialist, racist language.

Biden: Where am I? Who am I?

Harris: You are the front man for the southern segregationists who wanted me in chains.

Biden: Am I? I'm sorry. But I want abortion for everyone. Does that help?

Booker: Not unless you want it federally funded for all undocumented migrants, including those that are transgendered.

Biden: Is this where I raise my hand?

Sanders: Can't I get a word in here? We need to tax the 1 percent at 90 percent or more to fund free universal education from pre-school through graduate school, including at all Ivy League institutions.

Buttigieg: I went to an Ivy League college, I think.

Harris: Just because the former Vice President wants free abortions for everyone doesn't mean he has repudiated his racist past.

DeBlasio: Are we talking abortion now? I want party-selective abortions, only the fetuses of Republican parents.

Beto: Yes, but one parent can be No Party Preference as long as the other one is Republican.

Warren: We need economic justice in this country. Free month-long vacations on a Carnival cruise for all Americans earning less than $100,000. We will pay for it with a wealth tax on everyone earning more than $100,000.

Sanders: I wish I had thought of that.

Castro: Migrants are America's future. They must be treated properly. I propose a new tax to pay for Hyatt Hotel stays for everyone who crosses a border that shouldn't exist in the first place.

Biden: Now, Julian, that's going a little too far. Wouldn't a Red Roof Inn suffice?

Harris: Once again, Mr. Biden is showing his racist streak, suggesting that the inferior migrants don't deserve a Hyatt Hotel stay.

Klobuchar: I'm from Minnesota

Biden: Isn't that where Mary Tyler Moore was always losing her hat?

Beto: You see how ancient he is, he still remembers the Mary Tyler Moore show.

Buttigieg: Can we stop talking about age and instead how lovely it will be to have my husband be the First Lady?

Sanders: I don't care about First Ladies. We need Medicare for All.

Biden: I think I'm already on Medicare.

Sanders: Well that makes two of us. But how about the other 300 million Americans?

Booker: What about them?

DeBlasio: Most of them are racists. That's how Trump got elected.

Biden: I thought the Russians elected him.

Beto: The Russians are racists too. How many African-Americans or Latinos are in Putin's cabinet? None!

Castro: I'd like to be in a cabinet again.

Ryan: Puedo decir algo?

Harris: No, keep your mouth shut. You are a white male. You have no right to say anything!

Warren: Can we get back to the issues, please.

Biden: What are the issues?

Harris: The main issue is that the former Vice President is opposed to busing.

Biden: This is true. I hate busing. Sometimes they don't even have a restroom. I prefer a plane or train anytime.

Klobuchar: I'm from Minnesota.

Booker: I hate Minnesota. It is full of racist white Europeans. And it snows too much. And snow is white.

Biden: Did someone say Snow White? Is she here too?

Moderator: And on that curious note, we conclude the third Democrat presidential debate. For America's sake, we hope there isn't a fourth. Good night.

IT'S TIME TO RECALL GAVIN NEWSOM

August 29, 2019

CALIFORNIANS ARE FED UP. THEY HAVE HAD ENOUGH. That's the conclusion we can draw from a recent Quinnipiac poll showing that Gov. Gavin Newsom's approval rating has sunk to just 39 percent. Elected by an overwhelming 62 percent of the vote just last November, more than one-third of his voters have now walked away in just a matter of months. This is a dramatic and ominous collapse in support for Typhoid Gavin, the godfather of the Dark Ages-type diseases now spreading through some of our major cities.

It's time to recall Governor Gavin Newsom.

For many Californians, the last straw was Newsom's recent signature on legislation providing taxpayer-paid health care to illegal immigrants. This decision will take $100 million from the pockets of our firefighters and school teachers, our waitresses and construction workers, our plumbers and truck drivers to provide free health care to individuals who have broken into our country and violated our sovereignty. As a compassionate society, we are already taking care of illegal immigrants in the Emergency Room – by law we have to do so. Governor Newsom wants to take it a step further and grant health care across-the-board. And, believe me, $100 million is just for openers, like every other government program. It will inevitably mushroom and expand, covering more and more illegals until it becomes a giant new entitlement program costing many billions of dollars a year.

Not only will the dollar costs of this scheme become unbearable but the consequences for all Californians who need medical care will be catastrophic. We are already dealing with a shortage of doctors. Many are leaving the practice of medicine because of the crippling cost and stress of complying with government and insurance company mandates and regulations. We are now going to dump hundreds of thousands more individuals onto an already overtaxed system as well as providing an enormous magnet to lure more illegal immigrants into our state. Less supply and more demand equals what, in basic economics? Higher prices and shortages. That's what we face if we don't act to change this.

The insanity of this legislation simply overwhelms the rational mind. Under Newsom's plan, an MS-13 killer could receive free health care at your expense while the victim could be turned away from his doctor's office because he's uninsured or can't meet the copay.

And this reprehensible new law – just signed a couple of weeks ago – is what sparked my desire to recall Gavin Newsom. As you might remember, we recalled a California governor not that long ago. In 2003, a grassroots revolt among California taxpayers led to the removal of Governor Gray Davis from office – and the reasons were less compelling than they are now, in regard to Gavin Newsom.

In addition to health care for illegal aliens, let's consider at least three other major issues:

Tax increases. With a massive budget surplus of over $20 billion, Newsom wants to continue raising taxes on Californians, from the gas tax to higher car registration fees to a water tax. He proposes over $2 billion in new taxes. He would love to destroy Prop. 13 with the split roll tax assessment, which will drive more job-creating businesses out of the state. Californians already pay the highest taxes in the nation. He wants them even higher.

Homelessness. Cities like San Francisco and Los Angeles are now public health dangers due to out-of-control homelessness. Newsom is doing nothing about this. He is permitting great cities to turn into Third World hellholes with disease, drug addiction, public urination and defecation. People can't walk the streets, and tourists and their dollars are fleeing. His housing plans are a joke. The homeless can't afford any kind of housing in this state; they need medical and mental health care and drug rehabilitation so that they can eventually go to school or get jobs.

Sanctuary State and Cities: Newsom is the Archangel of Illegal Immigration and sheltering criminals and gang members. He is violating and subverting federal immigration law at every turn by shielding criminals from law enforcement and immigration authorities and making our communities and neighborhoods more unsafe.

There are many more reasons to recall Gavin Newsom, from his opposition to the 2nd Amendment, to his effort to shut down capital punishment in this state in defiance of the will of the voters, to his support for shifting the cost of PG&E's mismanagement of our state's wildfires to the ratepayers. He is a political extremist totally devoted to imposing an extreme left-wing agenda upon California. The future of the Golden State under Gavin Newsom will not be golden at all, it will be a dark and dangerous future of skyrocketing crime, higher taxes, uncontrolled spending, deteriorating public schools, a collapsing health care system, and more handouts for those who have broken into our country.

However, with a new governor, we can again have the California of our parents' and grandparents' dreams: a land of limitless opportunities and promise. A new governor who will work with the Trump Administration to secure our border and end health and welfare benefits to illegal immigrants and cut taxes so our residents and businesses will stay in California. We can start by repealing the gas tax increase. Fix our schools by breaking the power of the teachers' unions and introducing parental choice at all levels. Solve the homeless crisis by enforcing laws against vagrancy and public indecency, while getting our veterans and mentally ill the help they need through rehab, schooling, and jobs. Solve the housing crisis by slashing the taxes, fees, and regulations that make it more expensive to build a house in California than almost anywhere in the country. California needs a new governor. A governor in the mold of Ronald Reagan. A governor who can reach across California from our coastal towns to our giant cities, from our farm communities to Silicon Valley. A governor who can communicate a vision of hope and opportunity to all Californians: moms and dads, your friends and neighbors and all those who are working two and three jobs to make the mortgage payment, pay the health insurance premium, or write the tuition check. These are the people who Gavin Newsom and the radical political elites in Sacramento choose to ignore. It is these people – the Forgotten Californians – who can and will "Make California Great Again!"

If you would like to help, please visit *Recallnewsom.us*

DEMOCRATS: THE PARTY OF RACIAL POLITICS

June 1, 2020

D EMOCRAT PRESIDENTIAL NOMINEE-IN-WAITING, THE feeble Joe Biden recently ignited a furious firestorm with racially charged remarks in a radio interview with a prominent African-American broadcast personality. In the interview, a clearly defensive Biden, who was unable to advance a clear policy platform to benefit the nation's black community, instead chose to insult the intelligence of listeners by saying that a black "ain't really black" if he supports President Trump instead of Obama's ex-Vice President.

In making that statement, Biden openly challenged the racial integrity of the more than 1.3 million African-American voters who voted for Donald Trump in 2016, essentially calling them "Uncle Toms" and "race traitors." This was especially insulting and derogatory to African-American males who gave about 15 percent of their votes to the President. In making this statement, Biden is only the latest Democratic politician who uses and abuses racial minorities – be they blacks, Latinos, or Asian-Americans to get their votes at election time and then advises them to "shut up" and eat their soup.

Of course, we all know the sordid and ugly history of the Democratic Party itself, a virtual rogue's gallery of racists, hate-mongers, white supremacists, slaveowners, secessionists, cross-burners, and lynchers. The Democratic Party was the party of Confederate separatism and slavery. After the Civil War, it was the party that resisted the 13th, 14th and 15thAmendments guaranteeing the newly freed slaves basic freedoms. It is the party that fought Reconstruction, the party that denied African-Americans the vote, the party that enacted Jim Crow laws and literacy tests, established the Ku Klux Klan as its military arm, and unleashed lynch mobs to hang blacks from trees throughout the South. Woodrow Wilson, the first Democrat President of the 20th century was a virulent racist who decreed racial segregation throughout the federal government and hosted a White House viewing of the pro-KKK film, *Birth of a Nation*.

In more recent years, particularly in the 1940s, 1950s, and 1960s, Democrats in Congress were the chief opponents of anti-lynching laws. Democrats like FDR appointed KKK members like Hugo Black to the U.S. Supreme Court and KKK members like Robert Byrd became prominent leaders of the party in the Senate. Some of the most prominent race haters in the Congress were Democrats like Tom Watson and Theodore Bilbo. The presidential candidate of the segregationist "Dixiecrat" Party in 1948 was the Democrat governor of South Carolina, Strom Thurmond. Adlai Stevenson named segregationist John Sparkman as his vice-presidential running mate in 1952 and embraced the anti-civil rights "Southern Manifesto" in his rematch with Eisenhower four years later. LBJ led the opposition to the Civil Rights Act of 1957 – sponsored by Republican President Dwight Eisenhower. The chief opposition and most of the votes against the 1964 Civil Rights Act and the 1965 Voting Rights Act came not from Republicans, but from Democrats, Senators like Eastland, Stennis, Fulbright, and Gore. The governors who tried to prevent the integration of schools were Democrats like Orval Faubus of Arkansas, Lester Maddox of Georgia, and George Wallace of Alabama.

With a record like that, is it any surprise that the Democratic Party is about to nominate an individual who defended segregation well into the 1970s and associated with the Southern segregationist senators like Eastland and Talmadge?

Is it any surprise that Biden boasted that his home state of Delaware was a "slave state" and applauded locking up thousands of African-Americans in the Clinton Crime Bill?

Is it any wonder that African-Americans voted overwhelmingly Republican from the post-Civil War era until the early 1960s, with Richard Nixon still netting almost a third of the black vote against Kennedy in 1960?

Apologists for the Democratic Party ignore the party's vile past and instead claim that the party changed in the 1960s when President Johnson secured the passage of the landmark Civil Rights Act. The truth is that President Kennedy was lukewarm at best to civil rights and had to be pushed hard to introduce such legislation in Congress before he was assassinated in Dallas in 1963. The corrupt politician LBJ, who had previously opposed every piece of civil rights legislation, cynically embraced the 1964 bill as a way to "buy off" a new constituency with his "War on Poverty" welfare programs, which resulted in the destruction of the African-American family in America. Johnson figured it would be easier to ensure his party's future success at the polls by creating an underclass dependent on the federal government for sustenance and survival.

Such began the "new era" of the Democratic Party's policy toward racial minorities, not creating jobs, businesses, or wealth to make blacks, browns, and Asians self-sufficient and independent, but to keep them "down on the plantation" with AFDC, food stamps, section 8 housing, and Medicaid. Only under Republican Presidents like Nixon and Reagan did the U.S. government try to encourage the development and expansion of minority-owned businesses such as Nixon's "black capitalism" and Reagan's inner-city "enterprise zones."

Unfortunately, too many self-appointed so-called "leaders" of the African-American community, like Jesse Jackson and Al Sharpton, became little more than hustlers for the Democratic Party, willing to keep their people in bondage to Big Government to receive special favors from government and laudatory praise from the left-wing news media. They eagerly traded the votes of their community for crumbs from Washington and a seat at the table of a party that has always sought their enslavement. That's why when African-Americans like Tom Sowell, Walter Williams, and Justice Clarence Thomas arrived on the scene and challenged the "new plantation" agenda of the Democratic Party, they were and are vilified and crucified by the "thought police" of the Left, which will fight to the death for your right to agree with them and with them alone.

Joe Biden has to engage in racially inflammatory language in his campaign because neither he nor his party have any program to help African-Americans. Their "Great Society" programs spent trillions and failed miserably, leading to record numbers of broken families, illegitimate births, drug abuse, and crime. On the other hand, President Trump has worked hard to empower minorities in America, through record job creation in the pre-COVID period, record low unemployment, criminal justice reform, school choice, and opportunity zones.

Minorities in America are sick and tired of being stereotyped and pigeonholed by Democrat politicians. They are sick and tired of being used. African-Americans and Latinos want the same things as white Americans: liberty, opportunity, and the ability to raise and educate their families in a prosperous society. Instead, the Democrats offer them welfare checks, crime-infested cities, and sub-standard public schools. As Richard Nixon said in 1968 in his acceptance speech at the Republican National Convention, the Democratic Party's agenda toward the minority child is one that that "feeds his stomach and starves his soul. It breaks his heart." A half-century later, a truer and sadder commentary on the so-called "party of compassion" could not be made.

WOULD JFK RECOGNIZE HIS PARTY?

September 8, 2020

For three generations, John F. Kennedy has been one of the greatest and most venerated heroes of the Democratic Party. Countless leaders and luminaries of that party came of age during Camelot or drew their inspiration from him. He certainly ranks with FDR as the most dominant political figure of the party in the 20th century. His tragic assassination in Dallas in 1963 only raised his posture and position in the pantheon of American politics to near that of a demi-god to many.

Yet, what would JFK say about his party today? What would he say about the party of Bernie Sanders, Kamala Harris, AOC and last but always least, Sleepy Joe Biden? Would he even recognize the militant revolutionary socialist movement now masquerading as a legitimate American political party as the party of his presidency?

Let's remember the roots of John F. Kennedy. Irish-Catholic. Devoutly religious.

The Catholicism of his family was of the pre-Vatican II variety and it saw in Communism the Church's most ferocious and diabolical enemy. The Kennedy family hated and loathed Communism, the murderous ideology that annihilated 100 million souls, destroyed churches, and slaughtered nuns and priests. What would he say about Bernie Sanders who spent his honeymoon in the Soviet Union or Karen Bass who praised and idolized Fidel Castro?

In fact, the Kennedy family was so anti-Communist that the family patriarch, Ambassador Joseph Kennedy openly questioned in 1940 (long before Pearl Harbor) why the United States should take sides in a war between the National Socialist killer Adolf Hitler and the International Socialist killer Joseph Stalin. He had a point. In the 1950s, Ambassador Kennedy was a financial supporter of Wisconsin's crusading Sen. Joe McCarthy, who led the much-pilloried investigations into Communist subversion of the U.S. government but was vindicated forty years later by revelations in the Venona Files.

John F. Kennedy himself embraced the anti-Communism of his father. When the U.S. Senate voted to censure Sen. McCarthy in 1954, JFK did not vote. His own brother, Bobby worked for Sen. McCarthy's committee.

As a candidate for President in 1960, it could be argued that he actually ran to the right of his Republican opponent, Vice President Richard Nixon. He criticized the Eisenhower Administration for not spending enough on national defense and for allowing a dangerous "missile gap" to develop with the Soviet Union. He excoriated Ike for allowing Castro to come to power in Cuba. He made it very clear that he saw the United States in a clash of civilizations against a terrifying Communist foe. His inaugural address called on Americans to practice self-sufficiency ("Ask Not What Your Country Can Do for You....") and vowed to pay any price to secure the survival of freedom and liberty.

As President – though his term was cut short by the bullets in Dallas – he increased defense spending, confronted the Soviet Union over missiles in Cuba and over Berlin, and was preoccupied with bringing about the downfall of Fidel Castro and freeing the Cuban people. He cut taxes, the first President to do that since the 1920s. His Treasury Secretary was Republican Douglas Dillon. He was concerned about controlling the federal budget deficit and inflation. He believed in pro-growth economics, making him an early version of Jack Kemp, with whom he shared the same initials. He appointed judicial conservative Byron White – one of the two dissenters in *Roe v. Wade* — to the U.S. Supreme Court.

While he shared standard Democratic Party concerns about the poor and downtrodden, he was not the author of the welfare state monstrosities of the 1960s like Medicare, Medicaid, Food Stamps and the so-called "War on Poverty." Those programs were enacted by his successor, Lyndon B. Johnson.

When it came to Vietnam, Kennedy associated himself with the non-interventionist instincts of Papa Joe. While committed to helping South Vietnam defend itself from the Communists, he recognized that it was not America's war to fight and issued the executive order to begin withdrawing forces in 1964, not long after his assassination. He was distrustful of the "deep state" and wanted to put the Central Intelligence Agency out of business.

All in all, many of the policies of JFK could have been the policies of President Donald Trump. That tells us how far the Democratic Party of President Kennedy has descended into madness and pure insanity.

While he had his personal moral shortcomings, JFK remained to his death a faithful and practicing Roman Catholic. Can anyone see him embracing abortion to the moment of birth or transgenderism? Would he have encouraged the burning down of cities, destruction of monuments and statues, and looting of small businesses?

How can Americans who grew to maturity in the 1950s and 1960s and looked upon John F. Kennedy as a childhood icon now embrace the agenda of hate and nihilism pushed by the Democratic Party of 2020? How can they support a party that openly seeks the razing of the very foundations of the American Republic? A party that seeks to suppress free speech and freedom of religion and has more in common with Stalin and Mao than Jefferson and Jackson?

The answer is they can't and they won't. And that's why the Biden-Harris ticket is doomed to a humiliating defeat on November 3.

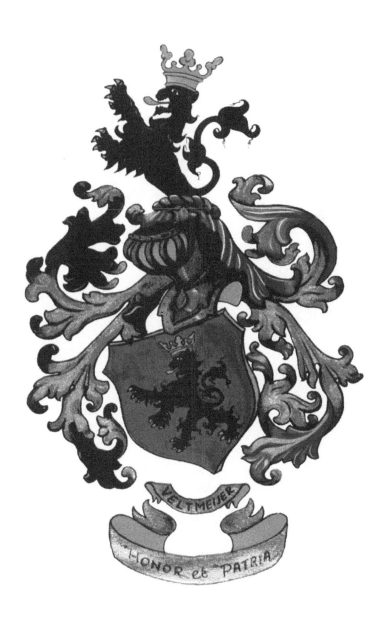

VELTMEIJER

HONOR et PATRIA

PRESIDENT TRUMP:

TRUMP: EXISTENTIAL THREAT TO NEW WORLD ORDER

September 30, 2019

T HE ONGOING ATTACKS BY THE POLITICAL ESTABLISH-
ment on President Donald Trump – which began even before
he was elected – are without parallel in history. The savagery,
frenzy, and outright hysteria displayed by the President's enemies
within the Democratic Party, the media, and the various power
centers of the globalist elites have no prior precedent.

This President has been spied on, lied about, made the subject
of phony foreign dossiers, insulted, ridiculed, scorned, mocked
and threatened. We have witnessed Hollyweird celebrities advocate for blowing up the White House, demand the President be
beaten, jailed or even assassinated, and his children tortured and
sexually abused. We have seen politicians in Washington try to
convict the President of non-existent crimes, investigate him and
his family members for everything from tax returns to guests at his
hotels, project on to him crimes that they themselves have committed, and seed his administration with leakers and double-agents.

No other President in American history has been treated in
such a shameful manner. Not Lincoln. Not FDR. Not Nixon.
Not Reagan.

What is it about this President that has roused such demons in his political foes? What is it about this President that drives his opponents to the brink of insanity? What is it about this President that so terrifies and terrorizes the Pelosis, Schiffs, Schumers and the George Soroses?

Is it simply that he is not part of the club, a brash outsider with a different style? Is it merely because he's outspoken and tramples on political correctness? Is it because he's sometimes unpresidential in his demeanor (at least in their minds)?

Not at all. After all, aren't these the same folks who loved Bill Clinton whose extracurricular activities involved cigars and staining blue dresses in the Oval Office?

Of course, Clinton was beloved by the globalist elites who pull the strings on world governments. He gave them NAFTA, after all. He gave them the WTO. He made tens of billions of dollars for them and their stockholders through these unfair trade deals that cost America 5 million manufacturing jobs and closed 60,000 factories. He also gave the military-industrial complex plenty of profit-making military interventions, from Haiti to Bosnia to Serbia and Iraq. Bill Clinton, for all his corruption, delivered the goods for the New World Order.

Donald Trump, of course, never played ball with these globalists. He was elected explicitly on an anti-globalist platform that put America first. From day one, he started to implement that America-first agenda, earning him the undying enmity of all those whose profits are secured by selling out American workers, American jobs, and America's national sovereignty.

President Trump pulled us out of the TPP. Billions in lost profits for the globalists.

President Trump pulled us out of the job-destroying Paris Climate Accords. Billions in lost profits for foreign nations like Communist China, at our expense.

President Trump began the process of securing the U.S. border. Billions in lost cheap illegal immigrant labor for the Business Roundtable.

President Trump imposed tariffs on China, becoming the first President ever to address Beijing's annual $500 billion rape of our economy. Billions in lost profits for corporations who ship our jobs to one of the worst tyrannies on the planet.

President Trump renegotiated NAFTA. Again, billions in lost profits for the cheap labor crowd.

President Trump launched the process of extricating the U.S. from endless foreign wars and avoiding new wars with nations like Iran and North Korea. Billions – perhaps trillions – in lost profits for the globalist war machine.

Is the picture becoming a little clearer? In each instance, the President's policies have represented a dramatic upending of the globalist agenda of both parties, the Clinton-Bush-Obama agenda of continuous war and the continuous looting of America's wealth and hollowing out of the American middle class. With both parties and their representatives in Congress beholden to campaign donors whose profits are threatened by Trump's America-first initiatives, is it no wonder that both Democrats and Never-Trump Republicans are determined to bring this President down? Most of the mass media is controlled by these same global corporations. After all, doesn't Amazon's Jeff Bezos—the richest man in the world – own the *Washington Post?*

As was said in Watergate, just follow the money. And while you're following the money, see if it leads to a $500 million left-wing slush fund run by a shadowy Soros and Clinton-linked group called Arabella Advisors which is funding the anti-Trump political agenda through dozens of high-sounding front groups.

The New World Order gang is in full retreat all over the globe. From Brexit in the UK to the populist governments of Hungary and Poland to the Yellow Vest movement in France and Salvini in Italy, the middle and working classes are demanding the overthrow of their nation-destroying overlords. The overlords who have flooded their countries with unassimilable immigrants from North Africa and surrendered their sovereignty to the European Union and its unaccountable bureaucrats in Brussels. They have lived the unfulfilled promises of the globalists, that giving up national sovereignty and relocating jobs abroad would usher in a new era of peace and prosperity. The exact opposite has happened. The globalist vision has resulted in $7 trillion of pointless wars in the Middle East, an immigration crisis, the loss of jobs, and declining standards of living.

In the United States, Donald J. Trump has emerged as the New World Order's most tenacious and determined foe as he fights the good fight for the American people, our constitutional rights and liberties and the sovereignty of our nation. He is an existential threat to the New World Order. Unlike other Republican presidents of the recent past, he can't be bought and has no price. Unlike them, he doesn't give in and he doesn't give up.

Go ahead, globalists. Try your impeachment games. Try your Senate trials. It won't work. In fact, it will backfire on all of you as – after three years of trying to prevent the Electoral College from voting for Trump, stopping the inauguration, unleashing Jim Comey and the FBI, CIA spying, Robert Mueller and his phony Russiagate probe, tax returns, emoluments, Kavanaugh, and all the rest — the patience of the American public is wearing thin. We aren't as stupid as you think. Something you will recognize clearly come November 3, 2020.

IMPEACHMENT: THE LEFT'S FALL FANTASY

December 11, 2019

A S THE DEMOCRATS' IMPEACHMENT FANTASY CRUM-
bles before our eyes, it is worth examining the actions of
recent U.S. Presidents to determine whether Donald Trump's
actions regarding Ukraine genuinely warrant removal from office.

President Trump is accused of trying to pressure the new president of Ukraine to conduct political investigations into corruption in exchange for military assistance. When one looks back
at recent American history, President Trump's actions or non-ac-
tions seem almost inconsequential in comparison. Actions of other
Presidents involved wholesale violations of the Constitution, military engagements that could have led to nuclear war, numerous
undeclared wars and even the seizure of private property.

Let's take a look:

FDR violated the Interstate Commerce Clause of the U.S.
Constitution numerous times with his New Deal policies. The
Supreme Court ruled so. He also violated the Neutrality Acts
passed by Congress in the 1930s. Was he impeached? No.

Harry Truman launched a War in Korea without a Declaration of War from Congress. He also seized private property (the steel mills) during the Korean War. Was he impeached? No.

President Eisenhower threatened North Korea with nuclear war if they didn't cease their aggression in 1953. He threatened aid to Britain, France and Israel if they didn't get out of the Suez Canal after Nasser nationalized it in 1956. Was he impeached? No.

President Kennedy threatened U.S. manufacturers with legal action and FBI investigations if they didn't roll back steel prices in 1962. He ordered the wiretapping of Martin Luther King, Jr. Was he impeached? No.

Lyndon Johnson launched a war in Vietnam without a Declaration of War from Congress. He tried to bribe the communist leader of North Vietnam, Ho Chi Minh, with a $1 billion TVA-style electrification project for the Mekong River. Was he impeached? No.

President Carter engaged in a series of actions that betrayed long-standing American allies, actions that arguably threatened national security, including unilaterally abrogating our Mutual Defense Treaty with the Republic of China on Taiwan (something the Senate had already forbidden and a federal judge later overruled). Was he impeached? No.

George H.W. Bush threatened Israel with a cutoff of funds if it didn't cease building illegal Jewish settlements on the West Bank. Was he impeached? No.

George W. Bush launched the catastrophic war in Iraq without a Declaration of War by Congress. Was he impeached? No.

Barack Obama engaged in a series of unilateral actions that were constitutionally questionable, such as changing parts of the Affordable Care Act without authorization from Congress and enacting DACA, which he himself said he lacked the power to enact on his own. He also intervened militarily in Libya without a Declaration of War and in violation of the War Powers Act. Was he impeached? No.

When one examines the facts, the realization that the current impeachment farce is simply a partisan political act to remove a President whose policies rub the globalist establishment the wrong way is apparent. It is also a calculated distraction to draw public attention away from the forthcoming Horowitz and Durham investigations into the criminal roots of the Russia collusion hoax.

If we refuse to impeach Presidents whose actions are expressly condemned by the Supreme Court or violate the laws of Congress or threaten foreign leaders with nuclear war, how can Trump be impeached for encouraging President Zelensky to "do the right thing." The truth is that encouraging a foreign leader to cooperate in ongoing corruption investigations or to reopen past investigations is hardly irregular, let alone a crime. Is it a crime simply because the Democrat's favorite senescent politician, Joe Biden and his relatives might be involved? Would it have been different if it had been a Republican politician's son who was implicated?

No nation has some automatic right to the hard-earned money of American taxpayers. Ukraine is no different. The United States has no treaty with Ukraine. It is not a member of NATO, even though it would like to be. It is a wellspring of public and private corruption. Not only is there convincing evidence that it tried to meddle in the 2016 elections at Hillary's behest, it was a lavish funder of the criminal enterprise known as the Clinton Foundation. Can you see why President Trump might have been a little suspicious of that nation and its government? Yet, while Obama refused to give weapons and other lethal aid to Kiev, President Trump is the only president to have done so. What more could he have done to help a nation with such a checkered reputation?

The Senate must shut down this Schiff sham as quickly as possible, but it should take all the time it needs to subpoena and put under oath the so-called "whistleblower," Adam Schiff himself, Hunter and Joe Biden and throw in Hillary Clinton at the same time. Let's finally get to the bottom of it all, rip the scab off this long-standing festering wound to the nation's body politic and learn just how insidious and pervasive this whole anti-Trump conspiracy is.

TRUMP 2020:
THE ROAD TO RE-ELECTION

May 12, 2020

D UE TO THE CORONAVIRUS CRISIS, THE PRESIDENT'S re-election campaign has been turned upside down and inside out. The economy has tanked, the stock market has crashed, unemployment has soared, and businesses have closed. Food shortages are on the horizon and trillions in wealth have been wiped out in a few short weeks. Civil liberties have been violated on an unprecedented scale. This bizarre situation has been the direct result of the complete and total overreaction of federal and state governments, misleading data and models, questionable advice from medical "experts" and hysteria stoked by the Trump-hating news media.

The President was misled from the very beginning of this so-called "pandemic." Going against his own usually correct instincts, he was sold on the laughable Imperial College model of 2.2 million dead Americans by the shifty Dr. Anthony Fauci and Scarf Lady, Dr. Deborah Birx. This led him to declare a national emergency and announce fifteen and thirty-day mitigation guidelines. These actions, which themselves did not shut down the U.S. economy, were used by power-hungry Democrat governors to suffocate their state economies and deny civil liberties in a desperate effort to secure tax increases, federal bailouts, or sink the President's re-election prospects. Others with more nefarious agendas saw the shuttering of the world's most dynamic capitalist economy as the gateway to creating their Brave New World of scarcity and want, based on the principles of the Green New Deal. No automobile travel. No air travel. An oil and gas industry in tatters and a guaranteed monthly income paid for by Washington.

What befell America was not the President's fault. If we were responsible for 320 million lives, most of us would have probably reacted in the same way when encountering a new threat and being bombarded with frightening death projections.

Fortunately, April 30 represented the end of the Fauci-contrived guidelines and that's good. The President now must now embrace a re-election strategy that will secure his political base and win over sufficient numbers of Democrats and Independents. It will not be easy because so much economic and financial damage has already taken place and it won't be reversed overnight. Nevertheless, the President should move aggressively now to move on from Coronavirus, allow the health care providers to deal with the problem, and restore America to some kind of normalcy.

Here are some steps he should take immediately:

1. Announce the dismantling of the Pence Task Force and its replacement by a new task force for reopening the economy and managing health care. This task force should be composed of free market economists and experienced frontline hospitalists who will ensure that the economy gets back on its feet while ensuring that our hospitals can handle any future Coronavirus flareups. An economist like Art Laffer or Stephen Moore should head it up.

2. Stop the bailouts and perpetual money-printing and demand the suspension of the payroll tax through the end of the year to help get businesses open again and employees back on payrolls.

3. Announce aggressive action by the Justice Department against state violations of the Bill of Rights under SIP orders. Unleash Bill Barr's U.S. attorneys on Michigan, New York, New Jersey, and California.

4. Take it to Communist China. Announce a series of sanctions and actions aimed at the cause of the pandemic: Beijing. Increase tariffs, repudiate debt, confiscate assets in the U.S., bar U.S. companies from doing business, return manufacturing, initiate a boycott of Red Chinese goods and reopen diplomatic relations with the free Chinese government on Taiwan.

5. Order a full investigation into the activities of the Wuhan Virology Lab, including the role of the ubiquitous Dr. Anthony Fauci in providing $3.7 million in previously prohibited funding for bat virus research there. What did Dr. Fauci know and when did he know it?

From a campaign standpoint, the Trump campaign should emphasize three main issues and hammer away at them day and night until they become etched inside every voter's head:

CHINA, CHINA, CHINA. The President must run squarely against Red China. He campaigned on this issue and has been proved 100 percent correct. Red China is an existential threat to our national security and our economic security. He needs to hang the virus around the neck of every Democrat who supported MFN status for Beijing, backed Beijing's entry into the World Trade Organization and allowed the looting of American wealth and jobs over thirty years. That includes the Clintons, Pelosi, Obamas, and

Sleepy Joe Biden. Expose Joe and Hunter Biden's financial ties to the Chinese Communists and Biden's lofty praise of that regime and endorsement of their aspirations for economic supremacy. This must be done over and over again on broadcast, print, and social media until Joe Biden is indistinguishable from Xi Jinping.

DEMOCRAT GOVERNORS. The President can hold the swing states like Michigan, Pennsylvania, and Wisconsin by campaigning against the tyranny of the Democrat governors during this crisis. Expose the economic and financial ruin they have caused to their states, their denial of basic rights like religious liberty and mobilize rank-and-file voters enraged by the actions of these governors behind the Trump campaign. These governors must be made the new villains and voters' distress over the economic collapse directed at them and at them only. Emphasize your efforts to re-open and re-build the economy only to be stymied by governors seeking perpetual lockdowns to increase their power, secure massive tax increases, and gain lucrative federal bailouts of their mismanagement.

SOCIALISM. The President needs to emphasize without hesitation the socialist nature of the Democrat ticket. He needs to point out that the temporary economic distress of the virus will become permanent as Joe Biden and the AOC wing of the Democratic Party put the U.S. in permanent lockdown through the Green New Deal. Campaign against Biden's promises to dismantle the oil and gas industry, ban coal mining, and enact the entire radical agenda of the Squad. Throw back at him his words that he's happy to have millions more Americans thrown out of work at a time like this to enact AOC's Green New Deal. He needs to focus on this theme in states like Pennsylvania, Michigan, and Wisconsin while highlighting the fact that Biden will return to "business as usual" on trade, shipping millions of jobs abroad once again. By the end of this advertising blitz, Joe Biden's face morphs into that of Alexandria Ocasio-Big Mouth.

The President, despite having the best economy in more than a generation hollowed out by the pandemic in just a matter of weeks, is in a strong position to win re-election. The polls show that. Having a corrupt poster boy for dementia as his opponent is a blessing. However, to win again, he must paint a clear picture to voters of the dystopian nightmare we face if a Democrat wins. The American people have had a taste of police state tyranny due to COVID-19, and the growing protests across the country are indicative that the American people will never accept the permanent surrender of their God-given liberty.

TRUMP AND THE LIBERATION OF THE REPUBLICAN PARTY

October 30, 2020

R EGARDLESS OF HOW THE NOVEMBER ELECTION turns out, President Trump will be recorded in political history – at a minimum – as the volcanic force who transformed and actually liberated the Republican Party from the vise-like grip of its globalist, pro-war, anti-national sovereignty wing. That wing of the party – except for a few exceptions – has dominated the GOP at least since 1940.

1940 was the year Franklin Delano Roosevelt sought an unprecedented third term as President and the Republican Party was in an ideal position to end the Rooseveltian experiment with big government fascist economics at home and interventionism abroad. FDR's radical policies had fundamentally altered the role of the federal government in relation to the states and asserted the supremacy of executive power over the other branches of government. Many of his actions were so inconsistent with the United States Constitution that some were declared invalid by the U.S. Supreme Court, leading to FDR's supremely arrogant plan to "pack" the Court with new members in 1938. By the time of the midterm elections that year, millions of Americans had experienced enough of Roosevelt and Republicans gained eighty seats in the House of Representatives and six seats in the Senate.

Ohio's conservative Sen. Robert Taft seemed the obvious challenger to FDR in 1940. However, Taft's refusal to accept the dictates of the Wall Street elites who salivated for the massive profits they envisioned from war in Europe led to the highly orchestrated but then totally "spontaneous" convention draft of Wall Street executive Wendell Willkie as the Republican nominee. Willkie, by the way, was the author of a book called *One World,* the very title indicating his globalist political philosophy. Needless to say, FDR buried Willkie in November.

1944 and 1948 were reruns of the 1940 race. Republicans again allowed the internationalist Wall Street wing of the party to control the nomination process. Again spurning Taft or General Douglas MacArthur, the party awarded its prize to New York Governor Thomas E. Dewey, a colorless candidate who offered no real alternative to the New Deal agenda of Roosevelt and later Harry S. Truman. Dewey was so hapless a candidate that he was easily defeated by Truman, who was given almost no chance of prevailing with his party bitterly split between its left-wing progressives led by Henry Wallace and its segregationists led by Strom Thurmond.

By 1952, a battle royale was emerging for control of the GOP. Mr. Republican, Sen. Robert Taft was again the frontrunner. Yet, the New York-Wall Street forces continued to distrust and loathe the small-government, anti-war Ohio solon. Similar to 1940, they sought out a popular figure that they could direct, an individual whose name was actually floated as a *Democrat* for President four years prior – General Dwight David Eisenhower. Despite Ike's wartime popularity, Taft remained the favorite of the grassroots. Had it not been for the downright dirty tricks employed by the Eisenhower faction to unseat the legitimately elected Taft delegations from a number of states, Taft would have won the nomination. Instead, the globalist elites won again and Taft was cheated of a long-deserved victory. It would be twelve long years of conservatives wandering in the desert before the Coup at the Cow Palace in July of 1964.

1964 marked the year when the first authentic limited government Constitutional Conservative in two generations took the reins of the Republican Party. His name was Barry Goldwater. While Goldwater would go on to lose the general election to Lyndon B. Johnson, he will be forever remembered as the political dragon-slayer who vanquished the Rockefeller Republicans at the Convention and placed Conservatives – even if temporarily and perhaps not consistently – at the helm of his party.

For the next sixteen years, an uneasy peace existed between the Sunbelt Conservatives and the Eastern Moderates within the GOP. They united to support Richard Nixon twice as Nixon saw the center of gravity in the party moving to the right and he campaigned to maintain conservative support through a strong appeal to law and order in 1968. The disorder Donald Trump faces today in America's cities is eerily similar to what Nixon faced a half-century ago as Marxist revolutionaries and thugs tried to firebomb American society and impose a nihilistic new order upon the nation. In the wake of Watergate and the collapse of the Nixon presidency, Conservatives were again ascendant in the party and launched Ronald Reagan on the road to the White House in 1980. The Reagan Administration was the high point of conservative achievement within the GOP, but planted like a viper within its breast was George H.W. Bush, heir to a Wall Street banking fortune, luminary of the Trilateral Commission, former CIA boss, and all-around reliable errand boy of the Eastern Establishment. Reagan named Bush Vice President with great reluctance to appease the still-powerful Wall Street wing, which viewed the cowboy from California with serious suspicion. During the Reagan years, a neo-conservative faction of ex-Democrats infiltrated the Republican Party, loudly demanding perpetual war and global entanglement. They became extremely influential within foreign policy circles in Washington, D.C.

By the time Bush succeeded Reagan in 1989, the purge of Reaganism in Washington was well under way. Hardcore Reaganites were sent packing and the Reagan agenda was deep-sixed as Bush began to re-tax and re-regulate the economy while committing America to endless wars in search of his "New World Order." Bush's quick repudiation of the Reagan Revolution led to his primary challenge by Pat Buchanan in 1992 and the subsequent third-party candidacy of Texas billionaire Ross Perot. When the votes were counted that November, the Bush drive to revive Rockefeller Republicanism had been thoroughly repudiated at the polls, with Bush receiving just 38 percent of the popular vote, the lowest percentage for a Republican candidate for President since 1936.

For a quarter-century after the Bush defeat in 1992, the globalists and neo-conservative perpetual war fanatics maintained control of the Republican Party. Every four years, they nominated a new member of the club, be it a Dole, McCain, or Romney. And, obviously, a second Bush – George W, an individual so devoid of any intellectual or philosophical foundation that he was easily hoodwinked into embarking on the greatest strategic blunder in American history, the trillion-dollar invasion of Iraq in 2003, and paved the way for Barack Obama's rise to power.

In 2016, Donald J. Trump tore up the Republican Party's dog-eared and dusty playbook. He vaporized sixteen opponents in the primaries –including the heir to the discredited Bush dynasty — captured the party with an army of working and middle-class supporters, and stormed the barricades of Washington, D.C., with the most unlikely victory in American history. In one fell swoop, he disarmed the War Party, exiled its partisans, and neutered its political agenda. They will not be back. The Republican Party has been permanently transformed by one man and the force of his unique vision and larger-than-life personality. The GOP has become the party of blue-collar working class America and there is no longer a place for the ruling class that bankrupted the country with endless wars and international entanglements, ceded our economic supremacy to Communist China, surrendered our national sovereignty to the institutions of the New World Order and threw open our borders to mass illegal immigration.

Many say that the Republican Party is now the Trump Party. In reality, that means the party has at long last been liberated and is now truly the People's Party.

THE ELECTORAL COLLEGE MUST SAVE THE REPUBLIC

November 24, 2020

THE MUDDLED RESULTS OF THE NOVEMBER 3 ELEC-
tion focus our attention again on the unparalleled wisdom of
America's Founding Fathers. When Benjamin Franklin emerged
from the deliberations in Philadelphia (ironically the site of
massive electoral fraud in the recent voting), he was asked by
a woman what government he and his colleagues had given us.
Ben responded: "A republic, if you can keep it!"

The Framers of our Constitution were students of history. They
had studied the ancient civilizations of Rome and Greece and they
were also fully cognizant of the flaws in human nature caused by
the Fall. They understood monarchy, democracy, and all the other
forms of government through which man attempted to govern
himself and subdue his raw, untethered passions.

Mr. Franklin was correct. The United States of America was
founded as a republic, not a democracy. The word "democracy"
is tossed around so much today by the totalitarian Left that most
Americans cannot discern the difference between a republic and
a so-called "democracy." The Left, of course, worships "democracy." AOC adores "democracy" as does Obama, Bernie Sanders,

and Hillary Clinton. President Trump is usually slandered as an "enemy" of "democracy" because he stands for the rule of law. The reason the Left loves "democracy" and the reason the Framers of the Constitution detested it is that it is, at its core, little more than radical majoritarianism: two foxes and a chicken debating what to have for dinner. The Left truly desires a "democracy" in which fifty plus one can enslave and terrorize the other 49 percent of the population.

Washington, Franklin, Jefferson, Hamilton, Madison. They all hated and loathed "democracy" as they saw such radical majoritarianism as a sure route to tyranny. You certainly have heard the term "tyranny of the majority"? That's what "democracy" is and it is a term that would be best expunged from our dictionary if we truly believe in the Founders' vision of self-government.

The questionable results of the November 3 election demonstrate why "democracy" is indeed the worst of all possible forms of government. In a true "democracy," a senile and corrupt individual in the pay of a hostile foreign government who barely even campaigned for the office can be elected President through a popular vote dominated by just two deeply blue states: California and New York. The hell with the other forty-eight states and their 300 million residents.

Of course, results like that are the reason why the Framers did not choose to have the voters select a President through a popular vote. They established the Electoral College and for good reason. Understanding history and man's fallen nature, they recognized the susceptibility of mankind to demagogic appeals that would try to manipulate and control the momentary passions and whims of the electorate. They saw that in ancient Rome and elsewhere. They wanted no part of that here.

Despite all the attacks the radical Left makes on this venerable institution, the Electoral College has withstood the test of time.

It is testimony to the wisdom of the Framers. It has helped pre-serve this Republic for 240 years. Its purpose was and still is not simply to ratify the popular vote choices of the voters in the sev-eral states, although that is how it almost always functions today. Instead, its original mandate was to be a "check" on the passions of an electorate potentially manipulated in their days by dema-gogues and charlatans posing as political leaders. Today, it should be serving as a "check" on the passions of an electorate manip-ulated by Fake News, rigged polling, and Big Tech censorship. Those three uber-powerful instruments of political brainwashing alone contributed mightily to whatever electoral advantage Sleepy Joe Biden may have emerged with. The Electoral College was designed to override the irresponsible decisions of the "mob" to maintain a republican form of government. It certainly has a role to play in a political crisis, as it did in 1876 during the Hayes-Tilden presidential contest when post-Civil War America was being torn apart by Reconstruction and federal troops occupying the South.

It can be convincingly argued today that America is in the throes of a deep and deepening political crisis. One in which, for the second time in four years, half the country does not acknowl-edge or accept the results of a national election. Just 49 percent of Americans believe Joe Biden was actually elected on November 3. Of course, at this writing, Joe Biden has been elected to nothing. And he remains elected to nothing until the Electoral College votes are announced in Congress in January. He is "president-elect" merely to CNN and the AP, which simply can't wait to herald Donald Trump's exit from the Oval Office. No, the Framers of the Constitution did not entrust the election of the President to a popular vote or to Big Media.

The role the Electoral College has to play at this time with this election is perhaps more critical than at any other time in our history. We are on the precipice of a Marxist revolution unleashed by one of our nation's political parties and backed by armed militias in the streets who will burn, loot, and destroy if they do not get their way. We are on the precipice of a technocratic tyranny to lock down, shut down, and mask down our country at the behest of global power brokers and so-called medical "experts" beholden to Big Tech. We are on the precipice of what the globalists call a "global reset," which is a euphemism for annihilating Western capitalist society and replacing it with a totalitarian socialist New World Order under the authority of the United Nations, the IMF, and the WHO. These forces – as Supreme Court Justice Sam Alito recently observed – are using an exaggerated health crisis to strip citizens of basic rights and freedoms and surrender their sovereignty to unelected Orwellian social engineers and planners.

The Electoral College must step in to save the republic. The red legislatures of Michigan, Wisconsin, Georgia, Arizona, and Pennsylvania must step in and assert their lawful authority under Article II, Section 1 of the U.S. Constitution to appoint the Trump-Pence slate of electors when they meet on December 14. They do not have to justify such an action, but can do so based on the grave crisis we now face as well as evidence of the massive voter and electoral fraud that took place on November 3 and 4. The Democrats' militias in the streets will undoubtedly be unleashed in response in our cities across America. President Trump can then invoke the Insurrection Act and crush the uprising just as Abraham Lincoln did 160 years ago. The stakes are too high now for the legislatures to sit back and supinely accept a Biden presidency. This cannot stand or the Republic will fall.

THEFT OF AN ELECTION
OR THEFT OF A NATION?

December 29, 2020

R ECENT POLLS INDICATE THAT CLOSE TO HALF OF ALL Americans believe that the November 3 presidential election was permeated with massive electoral fraud and the results cannot be trusted. Eighty percent of Republicans do not believe Joe Biden was elected and a not-insubstantial minority of Democrats apparently agree.

If these surveys are to be believed, America is on the verge of the greatest constitutional crisis since the Civil War. When one-half of the nation does not accept the legitimacy of an incoming administration and doubts whether we even have free and fair elections at all, the very existence of the republic is in peril. After all, what is the very foundation on which our republican form of government rests, if not the vote? If the vote and the voting system become corrupted and unworthy of trust, that entire foundation collapses and with it, America itself.

We are moving swiftly, inexorably from the theft of an election to the theft of a nation.

One of the nation's two major political parties is not a political party at all anymore. It is a ruthless and vindictive Mafia-like syndicate with violent street mobs called Antifa and BLM at its disposal to intimidate and threaten dissenters. It no longer believes in the Constitution or the Bill of Rights. It would abolish the First and Second Amendments outright and let the others die a slow, painful death. This party supports political censorship, the suppression of religious freedom, and the subjugation of the educational system to a radical, nihilistic ideology. This party worships raw power and exercises that power expansively as it uses a virus to confine tens of millions of Americans to house arrest, closes their churches and shuts down their businesses. Many of this party's leaders are paid agents and admirers of a hostile foreign power – Communist China – and it can be convincingly argued that they are guilty of treason.

Why should a party that now demonstrates – openly and defiantly – that it is indeed committed to the overthrow of our system of government even permitted to function as a legitimate political party? Back in the 1950s, many Americans fought to outlaw parties and organizations, such as the Communist Party, which were dedicated to the destruction of our republican form of government and were on the payroll of an enemy nation: the Soviet Union.

Is it any different today? Is a Democratic Party that spent four years attempting through every possible criminal maneuver to overthrow the duly elected government of President Donald J. Trump any less seditious than Gus Hall and his gang of Marxist thugs in the 1950s and 1960s?

Now, America is at the precipice. A paid agent of Communist China whose entire family is awash in bribery, kickbacks, and influence-peddling, an individual who is probably guilty of treason and could not even secure a normal security clearance in more rational times, has cheated his way – potentially—to the presidency of the United States.

The Democratic Party has no peer when it comes to cheating, chicanery, criminality, and corruption. It is basically a RICO operation. In 2020, they embarked — as Joe Biden himself admitted in a moment of senescent honesty – on building the most extensive "voter fraud" organization in U.S. history. Starting with illegally changing election laws in the swing states to allow mail-in ballots to be distributed regardless of eligibility to vote, signature matches, postmarks, or dates, they orchestrated the steal of the millennium. Added to that, they resurrected the tactics of Mayor Daley and LBJ to enable the dead to vote and the living to vote multiple times at different addresses and from different states. Then they moved to stop ballot-counting as President Trump led comfortably in all the battleground states and arranged for convenient late-night ballot drops of massive numbers for Biden –when the poll-watchers were already gone. Then they manufactured ballots from Communist China — pristine and unfolded— with Biden and only Biden marked and had them shipped from one state to the next. If that wasn't enough, they told county clerks to backdate late-received ballots and alter ballot information. And, finally, they made sure that electronic voting machines were rigged to "flip" ballots from Biden to Trump when needed, 68 percent in Antrim County, Michigan alone.

Not even an organization with the Roman efficiency of the Cosa Nostra could have pulled off such a heist. This required planning and organization rivaling the Normandy landing.

And, of course, just like the Mafia had dozens of judges and politicians in its pocket, the Democratic Party has plenty of judges who are equally corrupt and turned a blind eye to the Trump campaign's demands for redress – refusing to even examine the evidence but simply tossing out lawsuit after lawsuit on technicalities like "standing" or "latches." And, of course, the DOJ and FBI remained AWOL as their Deep State leadership prayed for an end to that pestiferous presidency that sought to "drain the swamp" within their compromised and morally bankrupt agencies.

America is at a tipping point. If Congress permits the electoral votes of states that broke their own election laws, their own state constitutions, and the U.S. Constitution itself to be counted, they will have betrayed their nation in a greater way than even Julius and Ethel Rosenberg in 1950. The Supreme Court already proved that it long ago abdicated its role in our system and now just seeks to be politically popular with the Washington and Silicon Valley elites, only occasionally tossing out a slightly meaty bone to constitutionalists so they can say they really do have a conservative majority on SCOTUS. For, with the notable exceptions of Justices Clarence Thomas and Sam Alito, none of the other justices can be counted on to enforce the Constitution when it really matters.

Is it now the United States of America, Rest in Peace?

Tragically and almost incomprehensibly, it is looking that way more and more as each day passes from November 3, 2020 to January 20, 2021 and no action is taken to stop the steal. America's political institutions have now become so deeply ingrained with corruption and criminality, blackmail and bribery, that we may have no other option but to raze them to the ground and rebuild them from the bottom up. It is a herculean task and it is uncertain whether the American people have the stomach for what would be involved. It would require a revolution on a dimension almost unthinkable to most of us. Yet, if we are to preserve what Ronald Reagan called, the "last, best hope of man on earth," do we really have any choice?

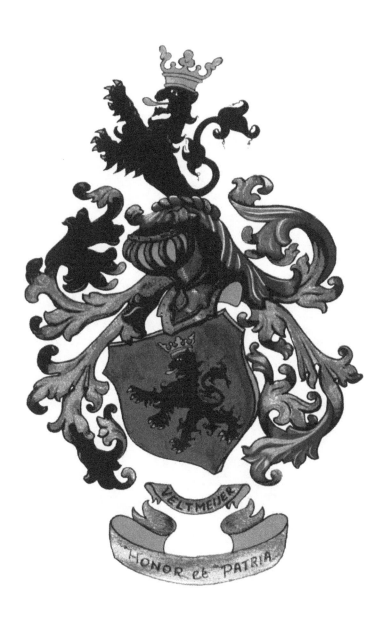

VELTMEIJER

HONOR et PATRIA

REPUBLICAN PARTY:

GOP ESTABLISHMENT: ENEMY OF THE TRUMP AGENDA

May 21, 2019

IT IS NO SECRET THAT THE REPUBLICAN PARTY ESTAB-lishment — controlled as it is by its corporate donor class — vigorously opposed Donald Trump's ascent to the Presidency. From the moment he announced his candidacy in June 2015, the GOP's ruling globalist elite felt supremely threatened by the straight-talking New York businessman.

After all, Trump was trashing all the fundamental tenets of the same party establishment that gave Republicans such winners as Dole, McCain, and Romney. He was calling for a border wall that would have denied the party's donors its steady supply of cheap labor. He condemned NAFTA-style trade deals that were dein-dustrializing the American heartland while enriching the donor class's stock portfolios. And, he was committing the unforgiv-able heresy of questioning the entire basis of the neo-conserva-tives' post-Cold War foreign policy, from unending wars in the Middle East to unquestioned support for NATO to uncontrolled anti-Russia hysteria.

Of all the enemies the anti-establishment political dish-breaker Donald Trump has faced over the last four years — from an unremittingly hostile news media to the coup-plotting Deep State operatives within the FBI and DOJ to left-wing activist federal judges to the culture-distorters in Hollyweird and the impeachment-seeking Congressional Democrats — perhaps his most damaging foes have indeed been within his own party. It can be convincingly argued that had the GOP leadership not worked so assiduously to undermine and sabotage his Presidency, Donald Trump would have enjoyed even more success than he already has.

Yet, he does have so many successes that he can point to with pride. From record low unemployment to rising wages and the return of manufacturing jobs, to a soaring stock market, energy independence, renegotiation of job-killing trade deals, originalist judicial appointments, historic criminal justice reform, and victory over ISIS. The list goes on and on.

Think of what he could have accomplished had he enjoyed the united support of his party, which held congressional majorities unmatched since the 1920s in the aftermath of the 2016 election. However, the GOP leadership in Congress was monopolized by Establishment swamp monsters like Paul Ryan and Kevin McCarthy in the House and Mitch McConnell in the Senate. Their first loyalty was to their corporate donors, not to the populist agenda of Donald Trump.

Illegal immigration is the classic example.

No one seriously doubts that the Republican Party elites love open borders as this policy keeps wages down and ensures plenty of inexpensive labor in the form of agricultural workers, construction workers, housekeepers, gardeners, and nannies. That's the reason the GOP has never stopped illegal immigration despite controlling Congress between 1994 and 2006 and again between 2010 and 2018, along with twenty years of GOP Presidents from Reagan to Bush the Elder to Bush the Younger. Republicans in the Senate like John McCain and Marco Rubio were part of the "Gang of Eight" amnesty advocates. Twelve Republicans voted recently to overturn the President's emergency declaration on border security. The GOP obviously places profits ahead of politics as uncontrolled immigration is on the cusp of cementing a demographic realignment in the U.S. that will make Republicans a permanent minority party.

When Donald Trump became President, he could have received funding for the border wall, if only House Speaker Paul Ryan and Senate Majority Leader Mitch McConnell had cooperated. They refused. Ryan, a shill for corporate interests, promised Trump funding for the wall but failed to deliver. McConnell repeatedly used the excuse of the Senate's misused filibuster rule to sit back and do nothing, despite the fact that he could have abolished the filibuster with a simple majority, party-line vote.

In fact, McConnell's adamant refusal to touch the supposedly sacrosanct filibuster rule (which appears nowhere in the Constitution) except for confirming judges was the reason that much worthwhile legislation coming out of the House never went anywhere. Suddenly, sixty votes were required to get anything done legislatively. Chuck Schumer and his merry band of Democrat obstructionists were essentially given veto power over the Trump agenda by McConnell.

The repeal of Obamacare was another fiasco that has to be laid at the door of Congressional Republicans. They campaigned over and over on this signature issue, but when it was time to produce, they could only lamely terminate the individual mandate and nothing else. This should surprise nobody. After all, the giant health insurers were the biggest fans of Obamacare as it forcibly corralled new customers and the Republican Party – like the Democrats – are heavily funded by insurance companies. And, again, it was RINO John McCain who sealed the doom on even a partial repeal of Obamacare with his infamous "thumbs down" in the summer of 2017.

Trade is still another issue where the GOP is at war with its own President. Donald Trump has railed against America's mushrooming trade deficits since the 1980s. His position in favor of fair trade has never wavered. Yet, this position that elevates the needs of Main Street above the greed of Wall Street made him an even more dangerous pariah among the party elites who profit off outsourcing American jobs and factories to low-wage Third World countries. They were outraged when he cancelled TPP, slapped tariffs on China, and threatened to tear up NAFTA. There was bold talk in Congress of overturning the tariffs and withdrawing the President's trade authority – something unheard of during the breezy "free trade" days of Clinton, Bush and Obama.

Even on foreign policy where one might expect greater unity within the President's party, Trump has been sabotaged. The President campaigned on a non-interventionist, "America first" platform that sought to disentangle the U.S. from perpetual war abroad and force freeloading allies like Western Europe, Japan, and South Korea to start paying the cost of their defense. Yet, even modest attempts by the President to withdraw troops from Syria and Afghanistan and pressure NATO to pay up elicited howls of protest from the "neo-conservative" peanut gallery inside the GOP. The President was accused of abandoning our friends, empowering Russia, and groveling to dictators. The "neo-cons" have dominated the GOP foreign policy establishment since the Bush era. They are largely responsible for the catastrophic wars in Afghanistan and Iraq, the mindless meddling in the Libyan and Syrian civil wars and the relentless saber-rattling against Iran, and remain wedded to the wholly unconstitutional position that it is the job of the American military to police the planet. Unfortunately, a top "neo-con" — John Bolton – currently serves as the President's National Security Advisor. A proponent of 24/7 war, Bolton is rumored to have torpedoed the recent Vietnam summit with Kim Jong Un.

As the saying goes, with friends like these, who needs enemies? President Trump must feel the same way with many of the members of his own Party. The President was elected on a populist promise to confront and take down the Washington political establishment and to unseat the permanent invisible government. Each day, he fought the good fight with some successes and some setbacks. Shouldn't the Republican Party have joined him, instead of working with the so-called resistance to take *him* down?

THE "NEO-CONSERVATIVES" AND THE GOP

November 21, 2019

O NE OF THE MOST DANGEROUS AND PERNICIOUS
influences within the Republican Party over the last thirty
years has been the so-called "neo-conservative" movement, a con-
stellation of scribblers, theorists, and political power-seekers who
are not conservatives at all, but rather, big government globalists
who have wreaked havoc in American foreign policy.

The "neo-conservatives" are actually refugees from the
Democratic Party who began abandoning their party in the early
1970s after the Democrats took a sharp left turn with the nomination of Senator George McGovern for President in 1972. These
"neo-conservatives" who started to rise to prominence in the Reagan
Administration (exemplified by then-United Nations Ambassador
Jeane Kirkpatrick) were old-style pro-labor social Democrats in
the LBJ- Hubert Humphrey vein. They were generally supportive
of the "Great Society" welfare policies of Johnson and backed the
Vietnam War. They may have been anti-Communist and cognizant
of the Soviet threat, but on domestic matters (aside from some cultural issues) they were largely indistinguishable from mainstream
liberal Democrats. They were not conservatives in any way, shape

or form. They were not students of Russell Kirk, Friedrich Hayek, Ludwig Von Mises, or even William F. Buckley, Jr. They were not with Goldwater in 1964 or with Nixon in 1968. In fact, amazingly, some – like Irving Kristol – had backgrounds as Trotskyites.

The Republican Party — trying to recover from super-minority status after Watergate – welcomed the partyless "neocons" into their ranks. That was a serious mistake.

Once entrenched through think tanks like the American Enterprise Institute, magazines like *Commentary* and the recently shuttered *Weekly Standard*, talking heads like William Kristol and Charles Krauthammer and foreign policy "experts" like Paul Wolfowitz and Richard Perle, the neocons began making their move to hijack and re-direct U.S. foreign policy toward an "all war, all the time" agenda. This agenda has resulted in hundreds of thousands of deaths and horrific casualties as well as $7 trillion lost in foreign adventures from Bosnia to Haiti to Iraq, Libya, Syria, and Ukraine.

The neocons had a particular interest in the Middle East. They even organized a secretive and shadowy group called Project for the New American Century to advocate for aggressive war in that turbulent region of the planet. Reflexively committed to the hardline settlement policies of the Likud government of Israel and equally determined to see American democracy planted and blossom in autocratic Arab soil, the neocons launched their first offensive in the summer of 1990 when Iraq invaded Kuwait.

It was never really clear what the U.S interest in the Iraq-Kuwait war was. Ambassador April Glaspie made that clear to Saddam Hussein prior to the outbreak of hostilities. The United States had no treaty with Kuwait and that nation was not exactly an ally. Instead, it was a typical despotic Arab monarchy with lots of oil. Of course, maybe the oil was the reason. The neocons never had a particular love of the Arab states opposed to Israel, except where the black gold was involved. So, when it came to the Saudis, Kuwait, Qatar, or the UAE, things were a little different and it was all right to send American kids to die for those regimes.

Although the neocons primarily perched in the Republican Party, their influence continued to dominate U.S. foreign policy under Democrat Bill Clinton where the U.S. continued bombing Iraq even after they had surrendered and new interventions were launched in Haiti, Kosovo, and Bosnia. Pat Buchanan once referred to Clinton's foreign policy as "drive-by shootings with cruise missiles."

Sniffing around for its "Pearl Harbor" moment, the Project for the New American Century got it on September 11, 2001 and within two years, President George W. Bush – led around by the nose by neocon Vice President Dick Cheney and his advisers – had the U.S. mired in the quicksand of the Iraq War. It was no "cakewalk" like the neocons claimed the war would be and no "MacArthur regency" was installed in Baghdad. Instead, the war devastated a nation, killed and injured hundreds of thousands, virtually wiped out the Christian populations of that country, empowered Iran, and destabilized the entire Middle East. By the time George W. Bush left office, he was the most unpopular President in American history, even worse than Nixon at the height of Watergate. Much of that unpopularity can be traced to the Iraq War.

Although Barack Obama was elected on a platform opposing the Iraq debacle and generally offering a lighter U.S. footprint abroad, anyone interested in peace knew the jig was up when Hillary Clinton was appointed Secretary of State. Called the "queen of warmongers" by Hawaii Congresswoman Tulsi Gabbard, Hillary's itchy trigger finger was ready for action from day one.

While not a card-carrying neocon, Hillary embraced the neocon agenda on foreign wars. Simply put, she was for them. Especially if she, Bill and the Clinton Foundation could make money off them. So, under Obama and Hillary, we lurched from one foreign policy catastrophe to the next, from the botched "Arab Spring" in 2011 to the brutal overthrow of Khadafy in Libya to the "red lines" in Syria, to Benghazi, secret drone attacks in Yemen, the 2014 coup in Kiev (which pushed Ukraine to the front of world headlines), to the largely discredited Iran nuclear deal. So much for the 2008 "peace" candidate.

The fruits of neo-conservatism are a world in chaos and an America whose National Debt now outstrips her Gross Domestic Product. A legacy of thirty years of non-stop war and turmoil, of using America's sons and daughters as mercenaries on foreign battlefields, and of failing miserably in their oft-repeated mantra of promoting "world democracy" and liberating the captive masses of the globe.

Neo-conservatism is not in fact conservatism at all. It has far more in common with the pax universalis of Democrat Woodrow Wilson than the enlightened nationalism of Republicans Ronald Reagan and Donald Trump. The GOP has never stood for the crazy concept that American democracy is to be forcibly imposed throughout the world at the point of a bayonet. It is quite simply a heresy within Republican ranks. And, like all heresies, it should be exposed and purged so it can no longer spread its dangerous and deadly errors throughout the party, the nation, and the world.

THE NEW POLITICAL REALIGNMENT

December 13, 2019

A MERICAN POLITICAL HISTORY HAS BEEN MARKED BY a number of political realignments that led to the shifting of party allegiances among voters and the domination of one party over another.

Today's two-party system has its roots in the Civil War when the Republican Party was founded to oppose the expansion of slavery into the new territories. After Union forces prevailed and the South was vanquished, the fortunes of the Democratic Party all but collapsed for a long duration. Republican Presidents and Congresses dominated throughout the post-Civil War era, with the lonely exception of conservative Grover Cleveland, the only President to have served two non-consecutive terms. The Democrats were almost totally consigned to a sectional or regional party confined to the South where its history as the party of slavery and rebellion was based.

Between Lincoln's election as the first Republican President in 1860 and Woodrow Wilson's election fifty-two years later, only Cleveland occupied the White House as a bona fide Democrat.

A number of powerful third parties also emerged after the Civil War, including the Greenback Party, the Prohibition Party, Socialists, and, most significantly, the Populists.

The role of populism is key to understanding the political forces now shaping America's destiny and its future. The People's Party of the late 19th century stood for farmers and workers against Eastern elites represented by the railroads, the big banks, and the so-called "robber barons." Many of them supported some very non-conservative ideas like inflating the currency and an income tax. In 1896, they united behind Democrat William Jennings Bryan who campaigned on a platform that promised to redistribute power and wealth from the ruling class to farmers, workers, and the middle class. He lost that election and two subsequent elections as well.

Republicans finally ceded the presidency to Woodrow Wilson in 1912, largely as a result of a split in their party between forces loyal to President Taft and those loyal to former President Theodore Roosevelt. TR's run on a third-party ticket all but ensured the election of the first Democrat in decades.

However, Wilson's election was only a short-lived revival of the Democratic Party's fortunes. By 1920, exhausted by war, high taxes, and inflation, U.S. voters returned to Republicanism, electing Warren Harding and ushering in another twelve years of GOP rule, only ending amidst the Great Depression in 1932. The post-Civil War Republican era ended after seventy-two years. A realignment had arrived, stoked by the deprivation and desperation of the Depression.

When Franklin D. Roosevelt swept to power in 1932, he brought with him commanding majorities in both houses of Congress as well. For two decades, Democrats controlled the presidency and with just a few exceptions, dominated Congress until 1994. Roosevelt forged a coalition of white working-class, blue-collar voters in the Northeast and Midwest which, aligned with the party's traditional lock on the then "Solid South" and increasing numbers of African-American voters abandoning their support of the GOP, ensured victory after victory throughout the subsequent decades. The Eisenhower presidency interrupted this in the 1950s, to be sure, but Ike governed in a largely non-ideological, bipartisan manner and did nothing to dismantle FDR's New Deal revolution. Once Ike vacated the White House in 1961, Democrats were back on top with JFK and LBJ.

However, fissures were starting to develop as early as 1952 and 1956. Many African-Americans swung back to Eisenhower and the GOP, enabling Ike to carry several South and border states that had never voted for a Republican. By 1964, the Democrats' grip on the Solid South amidst the Civil Rights revolution was slipping even more as Republican Barry Goldwater captured almost all of his fifty-two electoral votes from the deepest of the Deep South states.

Between the Civil Rights upheaval, the Vietnam War, riots in the street, and rising inflation, the Democratic Party was in a shambles by 1968. LBJ, who had led his party to one of the greatest popular vote victories four years earlier, was now presiding over his party's near collapse. Johnson's 61 percent electoral mandate in 1964 plummeted to just 43 percent for his hand-picked successor, Vice President Hubert Humphrey forty-eight months later. The combined vote for Republican Richard Nixon and populist third-party candidate George Wallace clocked in at 57 percent of the popular vote and an overwhelming 65 percent of the electoral vote.

The Nixon-Wallace vote in 1968 triggered a new political realignment that ushered in twenty-four years of Republican control of the White House with only the one-term sad exception of the hapless Jimmy Carter. Nixon's electoral strategy in both 1968 and 1972 was predicated on winning the South, now almost permanently alienated from a Democratic Party that working class whites viewed as more interested in appeasing mobs in the streets, draft card burners, spoiled college kids, and redistributing their hard-earned wealth to the undeserving.

When 1972 arrived, the Democratic Party lost every single Southern and border state. It lost union voters. It lost blue-collar voters. It lost the Catholic vote. Its base seemed to have shrunk to a bizarre coalition of hippies, left-wing college professors, radical feminists, and pot smokers. The old New Deal coalition of Franklin D. Roosevelt was dead and buried for good.

Throughout the 1980s, the term "Reagan Democrat" began to emerge as a term of political demography. En masse, former Democrats who were part of the old pro-labor, bread-and-butter, traditional values Rooseveltian coalition abandoned the Democratic Party and embraced Ronald Reagan and the GOP. This intensified the political realignment building since 1968. As the Democrats continued their leftward drift – especially on cultural and social issues –Republican ranks swelled. That realignment – despite Bill Clinton's capture of the presidency in 1992 – reached its full realization when Republicans won control of Congress in 1994 for the first time in a half-century.

Twenty-five years later, another realignment is in process. The election of Donald Trump to the presidency in 2016 represented a populist-nationalist reawakening among the American electorate that has little to do with political party. Trump ran as a political outsider, untethered to either party. He ran neither as a Reagan small government conservative nor a Bush big business Republican. He ran as a populist, hearkening back to William Jennings Bryan in 1896. He ran against the ruling class, the political and financial elites of both parties who had enriched themselves for decades at the expense of the working and middle classes. He ran as a nationalist opposed to foreign wars and globalist delusions, closer to the midwestern "isolationism" of Senator Robert Taft in 1948 than any contemporary Republican political figure. He turned politics on its head, single-handedly remolding the Republican Party away from its business-centered, country club image into what the Democratic Party used to be – the party of the working man. That explained how he managed to puncture the so-called "Blue Wall" and carry states like Michigan, Wisconsin, and Pennsylvania that had not gone for a Republican in a generation. That explained how he swept the nation's rural counties and dominated among those voters with only a high school education, previously one of the bedrocks of the Democratic Party. Hillary Clinton ran up her vote totals in the affluent, college-educated precincts where Chardonnay prevails over Coors.

Voters who previously saw Republicans as the "party of the rich" now see it as the party of the steel worker, coal miner, and truck driver. The Democratic Party has likewise completed its 180-degree transformation into what is now the party of the coastal ruling elites, the financial, corporate, and media elite of Manhattan, Washington, D.C., Hollywood, and Silicon Valley, ready to sacrifice the working class for crazy schemes like a Green New Deal.

Going into the 2020 election, the two parties have now become mirror images of each other. Few could have foreseen this even twenty years ago. The Republican billionaire New York business titan on the side of the little guy and the old party of the little guy now the party of Bill Gates, Jeff Bezos and the trillionaire class. Only in America.

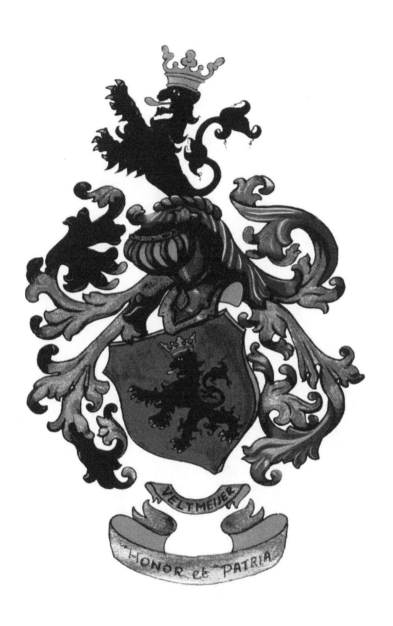

FEDERAL JUDICIARY:

DARE WE DEFY OUR JUDICIAL OVERLORDS?

February 5, 2019

THE BEGINNING WORDS OF THE U.S. CONSTITUTION are "We the People," forever enshrining the principle of the Framers' vision of limited government within the framework of a republican form of government, based not on the whim of a monarch, but on the consent of the governed.

Today, the question arises as to whether the United States of America is a nation of laws enacted by the people's duly elected representatives or a nation lorded over by a black-robed ruling class that enacts laws by judicial fiat.

Did "We the People" ever hold a national referendum on banning prayer from the public schools?

Did "We the People" ever vote on legalizing abortion on demand?

Did "We the People" ever cede to the federal courts the right to define marriage?

Of course not. Yet, these are only three of the many examples that could be cited regarding the modern judicial dictatorship that rules our lives today.

In each case, the Supreme Court arrogated to itself the role of our elected representatives and decided what the law of the land should be. No popular vote was held, no election took place. Instead, a simple majority of nine unelected lawyers was allowed to make law and the public be damned.

Is this the "democracy" our liberal and progressive friends talked about protecting from Donald Trump and his Russian election saboteurs?

The progressives shout, "Democracy, democracy," yet there is nothing democratic in a system of government by politicians in black robes elected by no one and empowered with life tenure.

The issue of judicial supremacy took on new relevance as President Trump, acting in his constitutional role of Commander-in-Chief, moved toward declaring a national emergency to stop the invasion of our southern border by foreign migrants, vicious criminal gang members, seedy human traffickers, and massive quantities of deadly drugs.

Even before he took such an action, political analysts predicted Democrats would go "judge-shopping" on the leftist Ninth Circus Court of Appeals and find a judge who would immediately strike down the President's action.

Yes, "Democracy, democracy!" If we don't like the decision of a duly elected President (the only elected official voted in by all Americans), we just find one federal judge somewhere, anywhere, to issue an injunction to stop him.

This is madness. This is the exact opposite of the constitutional self-government bestowed upon us by the Founders. This is tyranny, pure and simple. Yet, it is the preferred system of government of our liberal and progressive friends who have always seen themselves as an intellectual elite who know best and who "We the People" better mind, if we know what's good for us!

That's why the Left in this country has been misusing the federal courts for more than a half-century, treating it as a super-legislature to enact by judicial fiat what "We the People" refused to vote for.

We in California know better than anyone that the federal courts exist to thwart the will of the voters. Whether Proposition 187 in 1994 or Proposition 8 in 2008, the voters choose to enact their policy preferences at the ballot box, only to see a liberal federal judge immediately nullify their vote. Yet, this is "democracy," according to the Left. Their Orwellian manipulation of language reminds us of the many Communist terror states in the last century that called themselves "People's" and "Democratic" republics.

The truth is that the federal judiciary is profoundly anti-democratic and unless carefully corralled, it is the engine for the destruction of our system of self-government. Thomas Jefferson deeply distrusted the federal courts. He said they represented the "despotism of an oligarchy" that would turn the Constitution into a "thing of wax" they would "twist and shape into any form they may please."

Likewise, so too did Presidents Andrew Jackson, Abraham Lincoln, and Franklin D. Roosevelt distrust the federal judiciary. Each of these Presidents either defied or was fully prepared to defy a decision of the Supreme Court if it conflicted with the greater good of the country they were elected to protect and defend. As recently as 1971, President Nixon was determined to proceed with the Amchitka nuclear test regardless of whether the High Court ordered him not to go forward, as he believed the test was essential for our national security.

President Trump must be prepared to do the same, if necessary to protect our nation's borders and sovereignty. For if great Presidents like Jefferson, Jackson, and Lincoln were prepared to confront the highest court in the land, how much more justified would President Trump be in defying a lowly politically appointed federal appeals court judge who is arrogant enough to believe he or she should be making the laws for 300 million people? After all, is our system not based on *three* co-equal branches of government or as George Orwell might put it, are "some more equal than others"?

Mr. President, if February 15 arrives and no agreement on border security is in place, declare a national emergency and if a cherry-picked judge of the Left strikes you down, please strike him down, on behalf of "We the People" who demand an end to the rule of black-robed despots.

A POLARIZED AMERICA AND THE FOURTEENTH AMENDMENT

January 23, 2020

A S WE ENTER A NEW DECADE, A DEEPLY AND DESPER-
ately divided America is in danger of shattering along
numerous artificially constructed fault lines, such as race, religion,
ethnicity, gender, and sexual identity. Polarization of this kind has
not been seen since the late 1960s or even just prior to the Civil
War. Increasingly and sadly, we seem to be the Divided States of
America, rather than the United States of America.

Could it be that much of the responsibility for this polarization should be laid at the doorstep of a few lines in one section of
an Amendment to the U.S. Constitution ratified 150 years ago?
Could it be that this one Amendment has been misconstrued and
misinterpreted to spawn an "entitlement" society overrun by identity politics and groups and blocs of every stripe and strain all
clamoring for their "rights," often at the expense of the rights
of others – leading to a nation afflicted by warring factions and
burning hatreds?

It is hard to think of one Amendment to the Constitution that
has had more to do with the divisiveness we face today than the
Fourteenth Amendment ratified in 1868, three years after the Civil

War. And one section in particular has been most problematic. "Nor shall any State deprive any person of life, liberty, or property, without due process of law" appears toward the end of Section 1 of that Amendment.

On first reading, it sounds rather innocuous. After all, don't we all want to ensure that no man or woman has his life or property stripped from him because of the whim of a treacherous tyrant? Don't we all want to ensure a fair judicial proceeding or trial, the right to have counsel, call witnesses, and engage in cross-examination? Don't we all want to argue our case in front of a judge or jury? Isn't that what "due process of law" means? Yes, exactly. That's called *procedural due process* and it is enshrined in both the Fifth and Fourteenth Amendments, the latter simply making it applicable against the states due to the aftermath of slavery and the Civil War.

We must recall the context in which all the so-called "Civil War Amendments" were passed. They were enacted after the bloodiest war ever fought on American soil, brother against brother – a fratricide of hellish dimensions. Why were they inserted into the Constitution? The primary and some would argue sole purpose was to protect the rights of the newly freed slaves. They were enacted to give African-Americans the full protection of the nation's laws – even by the states the Bill of Rights did not apply to at that time (at least in the interpretation of the courts). These Amendments, including the Fourteenth, were not designed to protect the rights of women, ethnic minorities, illegal immigrants, homosexuals, or transgenders – as laudatory as the protection of the rights of those groups might be. The Framers of the Fourteenth would be dumbfounded to find this Amendment being used to "discover" a right to an abortion or to homosexual "marriage."

Yet, it all comes back to that troublesome little phrase "Due process of law." While you and I and the original authors of the

Amendment understand it to mean what we refer to as *procedural due process* – a jury trial, right to call witnesses, etc., some clever judges along the way had some different ideas. They came up with something called *substantive due process*, which is what it implies – it seeks to pour something of substance into the words "due process" like certain "rights."

Now, *substantive due process* has a rather ugly history, one which the advocates of judicial supremacy try to ignore. It was used in 1857, for example, in the infamous *Dred Scott* decision, to claim that the so-called "property rights" of white slaveowners were more important than the rights of human beings not to be held as chattel. This was eleven years before the Fourteenth Amendment, so this decision was based on the federal "due process" clause of the Fifth Amendment. Again, in 1905, in the widely discredited *Lochner vs. New York* decision, the Supreme Court tried to prohibit state working hour limitations as a "substantive" violation of the fictitious "liberty of contract" supposedly guaranteed under the "due process" provision of the Fourteenth Amendment. While the courts – in the face of the New Deal and Great Society revolutions that massively mushroomed the role of the federal government in the national economy—have largely abandoned the idea of "economic due process" as exemplified by *Lochner*, they haven't abandoned their zeal to rule by judicial fiat. Following the clarion call of the cultural Marxists, the courts started adjusting their *substantive due process* theory to embody identity politics, creating "rights" regarding race, gender, ethnicity, marriage, sexuality, etc., all of which have led to the current splintering of American society.

The great Supreme Court justice, Oliver Wendell Holmes, warned of the consequences of this twisting of the "due process" clause in one of his last dissents in 1930:

I have not yet adequately expressed the more than anxiety that I feel at the ever increasing scope given to the Fourteenth Amendment in cutting down what I believe to be the constitutional rights of the States. As the decisions now stand, I see hardly any limit but the sky to the invalidating of those rights if they happen to strike a majority of the Court as for any reason undesirable. I cannot believe that the Amendment was intended to give us carte blanche to embody our economic or moral beliefs in its prohibitions. (**Baldwin v. Missouri**).

Starting with the Warren Court in the 1950s, we saw the Supremes use the Fourteenth Amendment to find new "rights" for communists, criminals, and atheists. In 1962, the "rights" of non-believers trumped the "rights" of the 90 percent of Americans who were believers as prayer was banished from public schools. By 1965, the Court was peeking into the bedrooms, striking down a rarely enforced but legitimately enacted Connecticut contraceptive law based on "penumbras" emanating from other Amendments that have a loose association with a so-called "right to privacy" (which itself is not mentioned anywhere in the Constitution). By 1973, Justice Blackmun believed this so-called "right to privacy" (which did not exist) was broad enough to encompass the right of a mother to kill her unborn child. Shades of *Dred Scott* which elevated the "rights" of one group over those of another!

Whenever we cavalierly conjure up new "rights," we often trample on the rights of others. A woman over her unborn child. An atheist over a Christian. A member of a racial minority over an equally or better-qualified white American. That's why the Framers in their wisdom gave us a defined Bill of Rights, not a floating crap game. They gave us a legislative process and an amendment process which, while challenging and time-con-suming, allows for decisions to be made with deliberation and prudence with popular consent that will ensure that the rights of all are protected. Compare that process with one in which five lawyers on the Supreme Court decide on any given day what our "rights" are.

The misinterpretation of the "due process" clause of the Fourteenth Amendment has wreaked havoc and chaos in a nation based and built on the rule of law. It has bulldozed the rights of the states, destroyed the democratic process, invented "rights" out of thin air, and made us an "entitlement" society where various and sundry interest groups fight petty turf wars, demanding special privileges and special favors, all to the detriment of national unity. We need a federal judiciary that will consign *substantive due process* (which Justice Clarence Thomas calls a "legal fiction") to the ash heap of history and revisit any and all rulings based on this erroneous and dangerous misapplication of an Amendment originally ratified to protect African-Americans who had just thrown off the chains of their slave masters.

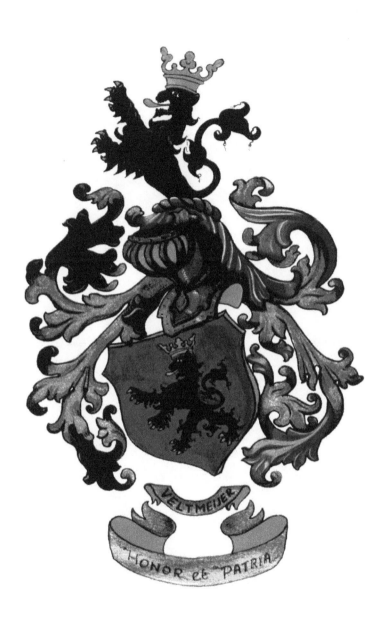

VELTMEIJER

HONOR et PATRIA

CULTURE:

MASS SHOOTINGS: SIGN OF SOCIETAL COLLAPSE

August 7, 2019

T HE TRAGIC SURGE OF MASS SHOOTINGS ACROSS America is neither the result of presidential rhetoric nor the result of lax gun laws. The Columbine massacre occurred on Bill Clinton's watch when the assault gun ban was in effect. Sandy Hook happened during the Obama Presidency.

No, the continuing explosion in violence in America—which includes the *daily* killing of innocents in large, Democrat-run cities like Chicago – is a consequence of the progressive abandonment of religious values and moral principles that are leading to societal collapse on a level not seen since the fall of the Roman Empire. These values and principles, rooted in biblical law and Christianity for more than 2,000 years, dictated a respect for the dignity of human life which has all but disintegrated throughout the Western World over the last half-century.

The embrace of a soulless secularism that can trace its origins at least to the days of the French Revolution all the way through the godless communist ideology of Marx in the mid-19th century to the Cultural Revolution of the 1960s has reaped a bloody harvest of death and destruction unparalleled in human history.

The irony of this reality is that the agents of death and destruction are the very ones who determined that God should be dethroned and Man raised in His place. That the worship of God should be replaced with the Worship of Man. And the result of their efforts in the 20th century: Two of the worst wars in human history, costing the lives of over 80 million people. The mass exterminations of Hitler, Stalin and Mao, which led to the deaths of over 100 million. Pol Pot's annihilation of half of Cambodia's population. Mass murder by totalitarian regimes throughout Africa, and on and on. All in the name of "progress" and creating a "new man." A "new man" without God.

This repudiation of the value of human life by the cultural Marxists and secularists in American society is manifested by the murder of over 60 million unborn babies since *Roe v. Wade* in 1973 – a holocaust of shame that permanently disfigures the face of America. And it is manifested by what we saw happen recently in Gilroy, California, Dayton, Ohio, and El Paso, Texas. For if any society can so callously and brutally destroy its most innocent and defenseless, what message does that society transmit to others about the value of human life?

Can we be surprised when a hate-filled killer in Texas guns down people at WalMart when the sitting governor of New York is given a standing ovation for signing legislation permitting abortion to the moment of birth? Or the sitting governor of Virginia endorses abortion *after* birth?

The tragic truth is that these killers and mass shooters are products of a society that has lost its soul. That has renounced its God. They are products of a public school system where a handful of lawyers on the Supreme Court say it is a crime to say a prayer. Where a Bible needs to be hidden on a school bus. Where explicit and pornographic sex education courses undermine and degrade human dignity and the moral standards parents try to inculcate in their children. Where "tolerance" of everything is demanded, so why not tolerance of evil? Where young people are even confused about their own gender! A government-run public school system devoid of morality must be seen as an accomplice in the acts of violence perpetrated by its charges.

If the public school system is to be blamed, so must the media—from Hollywood movies to violent videos and music to Facebook. Day in and day out, the media ridicules and denigrates traditional moral standards while idealizing the vulgar, the violent and every vice known to man. One yearns for the day of the Catholic Church's *Index* and morality code for movies that forced producers to develop clean and uplifting movies lest they suffer a boycott ordered by a tough Irish priest at the altar.

Sadly, our churches too have succumbed to the cultural Marxists, infected by an empty-headed liberalism that seeks to be in vogue with the modern world by abandoning centuries-old traditions and even the very concept of sin.

So, what hope do these young killers have? They are not getting it in school. Not from the mass media. Not even in their churches. And in many cases, their home lives have been ripped apart by divorce, drugs, and despair. In a sense, they too are victims.

Victims of a society that no longer recognizes God. And, when society no longer recognizes God, why should God still recognize society and protect us from the evil that contaminates the world?

Sure, we can ban some categories of guns. Yet, the killer in Gilroy bought his gun in Nevada and brought it into California.

Sure, we can strengthen background checks, but some of these killers had no previous record of mental illness when they purchased their firearms.

Sure, we can tell the politicians to tamp down the hot rhetoric. Yet does anyone seriously believe a few less Tweets from the

President would have caused these mass murderers to reconsider their heinous acts?

After each mass killing, we get the same old solutions offered by lawmakers who refuse to deal with the root causes of the crisis. It's just too uncomfortable and politically incorrect to say that a return to religion in society might be the best antidote to what is happening. Yet, as someone once said: "Religion is the basis of morality and morality is the basis of law." Or as Ronald Reagan once said, man has created thousands of laws over time, but has never improved upon the Ten Commandments. Maybe it's time our leaders thought about that.

THE CULTURAL MARXIST ATTACK ON WESTERN SOCIETY

September 22, 2019

AVE YOU EVER HEARD OF ANTONIO GRAMSCI? HOW about Herbert Marcuse? Or the Frankfurt School?

These names are probably meaningless to all but a small minority of scholars, academics and political theorists throughout the world. Yet, Americans – and indeed all those who treasure the religion, culture, and history of Western Civilization – should become acquainted with these names if they are to understand the forces that are currently tearing society apart.

Marxism appeared on the scene in Europe in the mid-19th century. Karl Marx and Friedrich Engels posited a thesis that capitalist society was doomed to demise as the "proletariat" – the working class – rose up to overthrow their oppressors, the "bourgeoisie" – the middle class of property owners. Marx and Engels saw world history through the prism of a perpetual class struggle between these two implacable enemies. Marx predicted that socialist revolutions would spring up throughout the West as the proletariat overthrew the bourgeoisie and established dictatorships in the name of the "people."

Fortunately for us, but unfortunately for Marx, his prediction fell short. The socialist revolutions largely failed to materialize in Europe or America. The Bolshevik Revolution of 1917 arrived in Russia – vanguard of the East – and had as much to do with the tragic casualties and deprivations of World War I as anything to do with the wealth of the propertied classes. Subsequent communist revolutions that attempted to replicate what Lenin achieved in Russia, be they in postwar Hungary under Bela Kun or Germany under Rosa Luxemburg, were either short-lived or failed altogether. In fact, the Bolshevik Revolution sparked a violent and equally totalitarian counter-revolution from the far right as Fascist and Nazi movements seized control of such European nations as Italy, Germany, Spain, and Portugal during the 1920s and 1930s.

Aside from Mao's communist takeover of mainland China in 1949 – which again happened in the East, not the West, and again on the heels of a major destructive world war—most communist successes in the post-World War II era occurred not as a result of a spontaneous uprising of the proletariat but at the point of a bayonet. Communist regimes were forcibly imposed by Moscow on most of central and eastern Europe as an Iron Curtain darkened the continent for the next forty years.

The intellectual followers of Marx were disappointed. Their vision of a worldwide uprising against the propertied classes – based on economics alone – had not caught fire. Their problem was quite simple: most of the working classes of the world desired to achieve wealth and property, so the Marxist siren song of hate and envy was slightly off-key. In addition, the communists' war on religion alienated the largely devout masses from that twisted ideology – a red flag indicator that culture, religion and patriotism maintained a strong hold on the loyalties of the lower classes and would not be easily overcome.

It was time for a new strategy. These left-wing academics – with names like Gramsci, Marcuse, Adorno, Horkheimer, and Brecht – collectively represented something called the Frankfurt School. The Frankfurt School – associated with the Institute for Social Research at Goethe University in Germany – was an assembly of political dissidents and malcontents who determined that Marx had gotten it backwards. Instead of an economic revolution igniting a cultural revolution, they believed only by a "long march through the institutions" of the West could they achieve their communist objectives.

To that end, they launched a broad-based attack on all the traditional institutions of Western society: the universities, the media, publishing, motion pictures, as well as the church and the family. Everything was fair game, if it reflected the traditional Judeo-Christian values of existing society – from sexual mores to national sovereignty. It is instructive to note that it was the very Bela Kun mentioned above who first introduced explicit sex education in the schools in Hungary during his brief communist rule, with the intention of corrupting the morals of children and undermining the authority of their parents.

According to the Cultural Marxists like Antonio Gramsci, a "cultural hegemony" of the capitalist class was using institutions like traditional marriage as an instrument of oppression. Everyone was now a victim of these cultural oppressors: women, racial minorities, immigrants, homosexuals, Muslims – it was the rise of identity politics embraced by today's Democratic Party that attempts to pit one group against another to achieve permanent political power.

As Gerald Warner wrote in *Breitbart News:* "By the post-War era the Cultural Marxist programme had a wide-reaching agenda of destruction. It aimed to destroy the family, denying the specific roles of the father and mother, and advocated the teaching of sex

and homosexuality to children; mobilization of women as revolutionaries against men, through aggressive feminism; large-scale
immigration to abolish national identity; dependency on the state
and state benefits; control and infantilisation of the media."

Of course, most Americans began recognizing the signs of
cultural upheaval in the 1960s, particularly after 1965, culmi-
nating in what Pope Benedict XVI called the "Revolution of 1968."
Suddenly, everything was under attack; even the very notion of
civil government and law. Authority was automatically to be questioned and anything and everything associated with the established
order and traditional societal norms and values, traditions and
ideas was to be wiped out. And it wasn't just in America where
political assassinations, riots, and college sit-ins became com-
monplace. Protests erupted everywhere from France to Mexico.

In France, General De Gaulle's government was nearly brought
down due to its insistence that students adhere to university rules
and codes of conduct.

Inside the Catholic Church, rebel theologians, priests and
bishops openly defied the teachings of the Church, a crisis of
authority unthinkable just a decade earlier.

In Mao's China, the Red Guards became the symbol of the
Great Cultural Revolution as they embarked on a bloody reign
of terror that rivalled Robespierre 200 years earlier in revolutionary France: killing, pillaging, tearing down and uprooting
every vestige of traditional Chinese society, religion, and culture.
Millions perished.

Cultural Marxism is the father of the Democratic Party's identity politics and political correctness. It is the father of transgender
insanity and racial polarization. It is the father of open borders
and rights for illegal immigrants. And, yes, it is even the father of
the anarchy and nihilism that gives rise to mass shooters and to

Hollywood movies that portray hunting human beings for sport as "entertainment."

Yes, Marx's economic theories may have failed, but his wicked offspring in the Cultural Marxist movement are having the last laugh on all of us who believe in a society rooted in religion, morality, and law. The fact that their "culture-first, economics-second" strategy is working can be seen in how the millennials—brainwashed for years by their Cultural Marxist professors in America's colleges and universities – are now so enthusiastic about socialism. It is this voter bloc— in addition to the exploding immigrant population—that the Democratic Party is counting on to stampede the voting booths in November 2020 to turn red states blue and elect America's first openly socialist President. To all of you who voted for President Trump in 2016, your vote is needed again in 2020, more than ever before. And, as one candidate for President put it in that volatile year of 1968—This Time Vote Like Your Whole World Depended on It.

A TALE OF TWO AMERICAS

February 19, 2020

A RE WE HEADING TOWARD TWO AMERICAS? ARE WE now engaged in a cold civil war? Are we on the cusp of national disintegration and separation?

These trenchant questions would have elicited simple responses and quizzical stares in the 1940s and 1950s when, it might be argued, America was at the zenith of power, prestige, and national unity. Most Americans asked that question during the Eisenhower era would not have even understood what the query meant. We were a different country then and a far different country now.

Just think back to that period in American history. We had just vanquished Nazism, fascism, and imperial Japan in the bloodiest war of all time. We alone held all the cards. We alone were the world's superpower. No nation or bloc of nations could challenge our wealth, productivity, or military prowess. Europe was in ruins. Japan had been atom-bombed into submission. China was in civil war, and while Stalin was advancing into Eastern Europe, the Russians had just lost 40 million people in the war and the rest of its population was locked in a totalitarian dungeon.

America in the 1950s was overwhelmingly white and Christian. Its immigrant populations of Irish, Italians, and Poles had successfully assimilated into the American culture. We spoke the same language, honored the same heroes of Valley Forge, Gettysburg, and Normandy, celebrated the same holidays, and, by and large, worshipped the same God. Families were intact, pre-marital sex was frowned up, divorce was uncommon, and drug abuse was rare. Prayer was permitted in the public schools and graduation ceremonies that did not invoke the Almighty would have been unthinkable. Abortion was illegal almost everywhere. And, even if it had not been illegal, it would have been considered hugely immoral. Hollywood's movies were clean and uplifting. Censors were not needed for *I Love Lucy* and *Father Knows Best*. Children obeyed their parents. And their parents obeyed God.

Was everything perfect? Of course not. No human society is perfect. Yes, we had problems, the most glaring being segregation and civil rights. Yet, even in the midst of Jim Crow, African-Americans enjoyed a prosperity unparalleled in human history. Black families stayed together. Out-of-wedlock births were a fraction of today's number. And, even in the South at the height of segregation, black and white children played on the same playgrounds and their mothers and fathers worked side-by-side.

However, something happened in the decade of the 1960s. It was determined by a handful of elites in government, academia, and the media that the America of Dwight David Eisenhower was bad, boring, or worse. Suddenly, we were told "God Is Dead" and that man was the alpha and omega of all things. That led to an insurrection against all authority throughout all sectors of American society. It was now okay for students to burn American flags and draft cards, to occupy college campuses and spew forth profanity in the name of "Free Speech." African-Americans were told it was all right to loot, pillage and burn down cities. The

271

Warren Court chimed in, creating new constitutional "rights" out of thin air, letting the malcontents and America-haters believe everything they were doing was just fine, a praiseworthy example of "dissent."

Those who believed in the traditional America of the 1940s and 1950s didn't fight back. They were what President Nixon called the "Silent Majority." Convinced by the elites that "intolerance" was the worst of all malignancies, they failed to stand up to those tearing America down. Yes, they cast votes for Republican Presidents, but those Presidents themselves lacked the will to resist the barbarians at the gate. They let the Left set the agenda, allowed the Left to demonize anyone who aligned with traditional values, and offered little but token resistance to the onslaught.

Fifty years later, the results are predictable. The fissures have widened and the divisions in American society have only become deeper and more permanent. Facing little opposition from the standard-bearers of American truth, the left-wing mob became empowered and emboldened. Constantly moving the goal posts, they demanded more and more concessions from us.

Abortion in the "hard cases" now became a right to third-trimester abortions, even to the moment of birth.

Tolerance for non-believers meant tearing down creches, menorahs, or monuments of the Ten Commandments, forbidding Christmas carols and abolishing Christmas and Easter in favor of "Winter" and "Spring" holidays.

A less judgmental attitude on sex now meant homosexual marriage and transgender "rights" to bathrooms and sports teams. Even pedophilia is okay in the view of some of their enlightened "academics."

"Equal rights," which promised to judge individuals on the content of their character rather than the color of their skin, was turned upside-down as "identity" politics took over, pigeonholing each of us into arbitrary racial, ethnic, and gender cubicles that would define what we had to think and believe.

A holiday for Martin Luther King now meant subsuming Washington and Lincoln to something vaguely called "President's Day" and tearing down historical monuments to any American hero who happened to be white, male, and Christian, from Christopher Columbus to Robert E. Lee.

It has now come full circle. The Left has never been more brazen nor has it been more bizarre. The leading Democratic candidate for President has staffers who want to put conservatives in "re-education camps" and execute landowners. Another candidate vows to give a nine-year-old so-called "transgender" child first pick for U.S. Secretary of Education. All Democrat candidates agree on free health care for illegal immigrants and most want to abolish the U.S. border outright. They endorse outright lawlessness as they embrace sanctuary cities and turn a blind eye to vagrants and drug addicts taking over the streets of our major cities.

Can you now see why some argue that liberalism is actually a form of mental illness? Does any of this make any sense at all?

We are indeed living in two Americas. One is what Hillary called the America of "deplorables": the smelly WalMart shoppers who cling to their God, their Bibles and their guns. The other America is the America of the rage-filled, hate-filled coastal elites, from New York and Washington, D.C., to Hollyweird and Silicon Valley. They are contemptuous of everything we believe and everything we cherish. They are cultural nihilists who wish to raze to the ground the America we know and build their new godless socialist utopia upon its ashes. They are the children and grandchildren of the 1960s troublemakers.

They hate the America of Washington, Jefferson, and Madison. They hate *you*. For fifty years, they have been getting almost everything they wanted and they have totally transformed America in the process. They succeeded because a series of feckless leaders failed to take them on. Until now.

This election will determine which America wins. The stakes could not be higher. In President Donald Trump, the Left has finally met its match. We pray to God he prevails again this November.

CHAOS IN AMERICA: THE SOROS BLUEPRINT

June 8, 2020

HROUGHOUT HISTORY, THE MOST DIABOLICAL AND depraved enemies of Western Civilization have sought its overthrow and dissolution through the sowing of chaos. Such chaos can take many forms from destabilizing economies to unleashing street mobs to burn, loot, and pillage. Perhaps the most outstanding example of such revolutionary chaos occurred in France during the 1790s, when Robespierre and the other apostles of unrestricted violence sought to destroy the monarchy and the church in the name of the secular "republic." Hundreds of thousands of innocent individuals who happened to belong to the wrong "class" were rounded up, tortured, and tens of thousands guillotined. It was so bad that it is popularly referred to as the "Reign of Terror."

The subsequent communist revolutions of the 20th century, such as those in Russia, Mexico, Spain, and China followed a similar pattern of murder and mayhem, death and destruction. All in the name of burying an "old order" and inaugurating a "new society" based on an extravagant egalitarianism that denied God, condemned private property, and saw man as subservient to an all-powerful state.

Mao Zedong's so-called "Cultural Revolution" of the late 1960s sought to wipe away and bury forever all forms of traditional Chinese religion and civilization. The maniacal Red Chinese dictator recruited and empowered tens of thousands of fanatical "Red Guards" to terrorize the Chinese population. Scholars, scientists, and intellectuals were killed or committed suicide. Schools were closed. Historical relics as well as artifacts were smashed, and cultural and religious sites ransacked. Massacres occurred throughout the country and even Communist Party leaders were purged and exiled. It is estimated that the "Cultural Revolution" resulted in the deaths of as many as 20 million people.

Another example that proves particularly instructive today is the May 1968 riots that targeted President Charles de Gaulle of France. In the view of the Left, de Gaulle represented a conservative, Catholic, middle-class *"ancien regime"* that needed to be annihilated. Starting with student protests demanding "sexual freedom" in universities, the unrest spread to communist-organized unions, leading to a general strike and the virtual collapse of the economy. General de Gaulle, hero of the "Free French" during World War II, briefly had to flee his country. However, in the end, the people rallied to de Gaulle and led his party to a convincing victory in the next general election.

The emissaries of anarchism and nihilism who represent the vanguard of all revolutionary movements have recently targeted the United States for civil disorder unseen since the days of the late 1960s, when race riots and Vietnam War protests engulfed a deeply divided nation. Capitalizing on the tragic death of an African-American at the hands of an obviously guilty police officer, hundreds of American cities have in recent weeks fallen victim to the revolutionary forces of chaos seeking to destabilize

276

American society in a presidential election year. These forces have taken over our streets, intimidated public officials, burned buildings, assaulted law enforcement officers, and wreaked havoc on innocent citizens and businesses still reeling from the impact of the COVID-19 lockdowns. What perfect timing – in the minds of sadistic nation-wreckers – to toss another match onto the fires of discontent raging across the land. In a just few short months, a nation that entered a new decade with a booming economy, widespread prosperity, and a future filled with hope and optimism, has been knocked to the ground and nearly suffocated, not unlike the poor unfortunate George Floyd.

Has it all been coincidental? Was the French Revolution just happenstance? Did Mao's Red Guards take to the streets just because they had nothing better to do? Of course not. Revolutions are seldom spontaneous, especially when they spring up all at once, *everywhere*. All revolutions require planning and organization and money.

Anyone who has studied the turmoil that rocked America a half-century ago recognizes the important role played by the Communist Party, USA and its various front groups in funding and instigating racial violence in our major cities. The CPUSA was, of course, lavishly financed by the Soviet Communist Party, and using race to divide and inflame Americans against one another had long been a chief objective of the Soviets. Likewise, the protests against the war were encouraged and promoted by Moscow through groups like the DuBois Clubs, the Students for a Democratic Society, and the Student Non-Violent Coordinating Committee. Many of the leaders of these groups were the so-called "red diaper babies," the children of Communist Party functionaries in the U.S. during the 1930s and 1940s.

Today, we are dealing with groups like Antifa and Black Lives Matter. And we know one of the world's prime purveyors of disorder is someone author Stefan Kanfer refers to as the "Connoisseur of Chaos," the Hungarian uber-billionaire and one-time Nazi collaborator George Soros. According to Soros, "The main obstacle to a stable and just world order is the United States." Readers interested in hearing Soros in his own words might want to watch a 1998 interview on *60 Minutes*: https://www.youtube.com/watch?v=QT_PGEG87m8

A ruthlessly shrewd international currency speculator who made his fortune of more than $26 billion by shorting foreign currencies and crashing economies, Soros turned his attention some time ago to a more sinister agenda, setting up organizations dedicated to, in author Kanfer's words, "social agitation" with a devotion to the "eradication of national sovereignty." Kanfer says that Soros' activities have "caused tsunamis of upheaval, in the United States and around the world."

In the U.S., Soros has been busy funding efforts to subvert the Roman Catholic Church, working through Hillary Clinton's ex-campaign manager John Podesta, who advocated for a so-called "Catholic Spring" based on changing Church teaching on abortion, contraception, and homosexuality.

He also bankrolls the radical left *MoveOn.org* movement as well as Black Lives Matter ($33 million in 2016 alone), stating as his goal the "dismantling" of local law enforcement. He has spent millions of dollars on political races in the United States, on behalf of "open borders" candidates and even local district attorney contests in support of "soft on crime" candidates. He has been a promiscuous backer of initiatives to decriminalize drug use throughout the United States. It is estimated that between 2009 and 2014, Soros' Open Society Foundations channeled more than $827 million to over 2,200 left-wing organizations in the United States, including those favoring radical environmentalism, wealth redistribution, abolition of the death penalty, rights for illegal immigrants, and abortion ($20 million to Planned Parenthood). In Europe, his activities have centered on encouraging the massive migration of North African Muslims into Italy, Germany and other nations.

An Open Society Foundations 2015-2018 U.S. Programs strategic plan that was taken from the group and leaked indicates that among other things, Open Society Foundations' U.S. Programs platform calls for:

An economy governed by the "redistribution of resources;"

A justice system that reduces incarceration, abolishes the death penalty, and promotes "health centered" drug use punishment;

Enactment of comprehensive immigration reform, that gives "full political, economic, and civic participation" to illegal immigrants;

A reduction in "the racial wealth gap" through income redistribution;

"Inclusive economic development" focused on raising the minimum wage and employment for ex-convicts.

There can be little doubt that George Soros' hand is behind much of the violence sweeping our nation's cities today. This has nothing to do with George Floyd. It has everything to do with another George, a megalomaniacal globalist predator who uses his ill-gotten wealth to subvert nations and undercut the rule of law. He is a mastermind of chaos, an enemy of all those who believe in the founding principles of this nation, ordered liberty based on law rooted in the Ten Commandments. He and his front groups should be investigated by Congress and all funding of internal subversion by foreign sources like Soros should be prohibited.

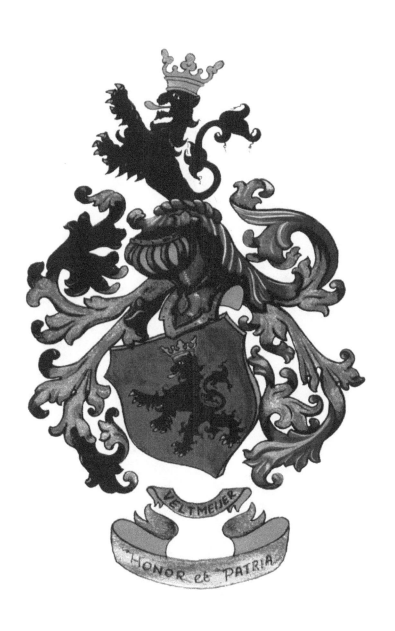

EDUCATION:

LET THE FREE MARKET SOLVE THE CRISIS OF HIGHER EDUCATION

May 8, 2019

1965 WAS A PORTENTOUS YEAR IN AMERICAN HISTORY, with a long-lasting impact on numerous aspects of American life decades down the road. For example, it was the year that President Lyndon B. Johnson committed the United States to a ground war in Southeast Asia with the unfortunate result of radicalizing an entire generation of young Americans and provoking riots and civil disorder throughout our nation.

Johnson, who had acceded to the presidency after the tragic assassination of President John F. Kennedy in Dallas in November 1963, had just vanquished Arizona Sen. Barry Goldwater in the 1964 presidential election, sweeping in commanding Democrat majorities in both Houses of Congress. LBJ believed he had the electoral mandate to enact his cherished "Great Society" vision of a paternalistic federal government at home while waging war on Communists thousands of miles away.

It was an ambitious agenda.

Yet, the consequences of much of LBJ's domestic policy agenda legislated in 1965 are concluding in the near-collapse of many of our most important public and private institutions in

America today. Health care, for example. In that year, the federal government injected itself into the lives of physicians and patients on a level never before imagined. Medicare and Medicaid were born, promising health care coverage to the aged and poor. While no one doubts the sincerity of the authors of these game-changing laws, there is a good reason why the American Medical Association (AMA) fought so hard against their passage. No, it wasn't because doctors were greedy (the truth is Medicare reimbursements to doctors are about the same as they were twenty years ago).It was because the AMA was prescient enough to see the effect on costs and demand that would result from the federal government pouring billions of new dollars into the health care system as well as the inevitable diminishment of the doctor-patient relationship. The fact is indisputable that the enormous rise in the cost of health care in the United States can be largely traced to 1965 when LBJ and the federal government jumped in in a big Texan way. Simple charts prove this, and Medicare is now within six or seven years of complete insolvency as it did what most Big Government programs do: overpromise and underdeliver.

Education is the other victim of the 1965 "Great Society" fantasy. Prior to that year, schools were primarily a local responsibility, controlled by local school boards and answerable to local voters. Funded mostly by property taxes, America's public schools largely adhered to traditional models of teaching and discipline and were — if not the envy of the world—certainly respected. As liberals can seldom let a good thing stand, LBJ launched a massive federal intervention into our nation's schools through the Elementary and Secondary Education Act of 1965 and the Higher Education Act of 1965. Both bills promised massive new federal resources to assist schools, teachers, and students.

As in health care, the results were predictable but even more negative. Despite Medicare and Medicaid, the quality of medical care in America remains high even if the delivery system is faulty. In education, however, the arrival of federal aid led to a quick collapse in standards, curriculum, and test results. Despite huge infusions of federal dollars, our nation's public schools became infested with crime, drugs, poor teachers, lax disciplinary standards, and embarrassing test scores. Students graduate from high school unable to read and write basic English. Entering college freshmen would flunk a grammar school history and geography test from a century earlier. Many can't name the three branches of our government or identify a fraction of the fifty states. Many are placed into remedial classes when they go to a university.

The situation in higher education has drawn much of the most contemporary political attention, with vote-buying politicians falling all over each other to promise "free" college tuition at public colleges and universities. Alexandria Ocasio-Big Mouth has supposedly even promised to make the Electoral College tuition-free!

Yes, it is true that the cost of higher education has soared over the last several decades and millions of students graduate carrying tens of thousands of dollars of college debt and can't find jobs for their degrees in Renaissance Theology or Hegelian Philosophy. However, is the answer really having a federal government, already adding a trillion dollars to the national debt every year, offer anything more that is "free"? For if government ever offers you anything "free," be prepared to hold on to your wallet.

The cost of higher education in the U.S. has climbed more than 538 percent since 1985, twice as high as medical costs and almost five times more than the Consumer Price Index. This increase correlates to two factors: 1. The increased availability of student loans and other assistance offered by the federal government, and 2. the increased demand for a college education caused by the ready availability of such financial aid. Let's remember the truism that if you subsidize something, you will get more of it. By massively subsidizing the cost of higher education, we have greatly increased the number of students and greatly increased tuition and fees, because when more money is sloshing around, prices go up. That's called inflation. Colleges and universities have gone on extravagant building sprees, massively expanded bureaucracies, and have handed administrators salaries that even touch seven figures. Yes, parents, that's where your tuition payments are going.

About the time LBJ launched his Big Government programs, the idea was hatched that everyone deserved a university education. It's similar to the Clinton and Bush Administrations' belief that everyone should own a home, which led directly to the subprime mortgage crisis and the economic collapse of 2008. The reality is that not everyone does deserve or need a four-year university degree. Not everyone is destined to be an anthropologist or a sociology professor. As a nation, we need skilled mechanics, truck drivers, plumbers, painters, welders, and electricians. Many of these good-paying jobs go begging because too many young people are chasing degrees that have no relevance in today's job market. We do a grave disservice to millions of young Americans by persuading them that they should embark on careers in obscure professions instead of learning a trade hands-on, as we used to do with apprenticeships. There remains more of a need for trade schools and vocational education than ever before.

If we are to fix the crisis in higher education today, we need to determine as a nation the inherent value of a four-year degree compared to one from a two-year community college or trade school. Where are the jobs of the future and what skills are needed to fill them? Are some degrees worth incurring a debt bill of $100,000 or more? We need to stop having government use its taxing and spending powers to engage in central planning of our lives, whether it's the kind of health care that's right for you or the type of education your son or daughter should receive. The free market has historically been the best vehicle for allocating talent and resources that man has ever devised. Let's give it a chance again!

UNIVERSITIES: HOTBEDS OF CULTURAL REVOLUTION

July 1, 2020

THE "LONG MARCH THROUGH THE INSTITUTIONS" IS A phrase popularized by the Cultural Marxists of the 1960s, who described their political strategy for destabilizing and overthrowing Western capitalist society. In no institution have they had more success than in academia where the universities today have become little more than hotbeds of revolutionary ferment and laboratories of political and social indoctrination. The radical overturning of American society we are witnessing in our cities and on our streets today – focusing on Maoist tactics of historical revisionism, cultural destruction, and public humiliation of political opponents – is a product of the stealth-like campaign to capture America's institutions of higher education, which has been ongoing for generations.

As far back as 1951, conservative icon William F. Buckley, Jr., was writing of this process of subversion of Western values in the universities in his classic book, *God and Man at Yale*. Buckley accused the professoriate at Yale of working to break down the religious beliefs of students and inculcate them with secularist ideologies and Keynesian and collectivist economics. Of course, the 1950s was also the high point of congressional investigations of communist infiltration into the American government and other key institutions. Not surprisingly, these investigations revealed significant numbers of active or former Communists occupying faculty positions in colleges and universities across the U.S.

The leftist revolutionaries who sparked uprisings on American campuses throughout the 1960s, from the "Filthy Speech Movement" at Berkeley to the actual takeover of university buildings at Columbia in 1968, sadly represented the future of higher education in America in the subsequent decades. While conservative students generally went into law, medicine or business to make a difference or make money, the generation of "red diaper babies" saw an opportunity to cause trouble, shape innocent minds, and impose extremist ideologies upon a new generation of vulnerable young people, particularly those who entered college without any deep-seated religious, moral, or political views formed in the home.

With the administration of the universities undoubtedly cowed by the terrifying events of the 1960s (a notable exception being the plucky tam o'shanter-wearing S.I. Hayakawa at San Francisco State University), there was easy entry into the faculty lounges at America's most prestigious academies. The left-wing ideologues made their move on the political science, history, sociology, liberal arts, and humanities departments. With a patient and gradualist strategy that would make the most dedicated member of the Fabian Society proud, they went to work.

First, we saw the demands for more "inclusive" curricula, demanding courses in "ethnic studies," "Chicano studies," and the like. These were innocuously offered as examples of "academic freedom" and gaining a broader view of American history. From that position, it wasn't much of a leap to begin challenging the content or even the existence of courses in Western Civilization.

We can all recall Jesse Jackson leading the demonstrations at Stanford in the late 1980s, shouting "Hey, hey, ho, ho, Western Civ has got to go..." From that point forward, we knew that the Cultural Marxists seizing the reins at Harvard, Princeton, and Yale weren't simply seeking to expose students to "new" ideas, they were trying to tear down our very culture and our very history.

Soon after, we started hearing about "political correctness" in which ideas which did not conform to the dictum of the reigning left-wing thought police in the universities were to be first ridiculed and then silenced. So much for "academic freedom" and the "right" of dissent as conservative authors and speakers were chased from college campuses, shouted down or even physically assaulted. Conservative and Republican college organizations found their ability to get chartered and organized being stifled. Next, we learned of "speech codes" and "speech zones" where students' First Amendment rights were severely restricted, especially if it was conservative speech. Students who disagreed politically with their professors were forced to remain silent or have their grades marked down. A totalitarian Iron Curtain had descended on the Ivy League.

Next, they came for our holidays and our heroes. Christmas vacation was abolished in favor of "Winter Break" and Easter vacation was eliminated in favor of "Spring Break" so that college kids could run to Florida to get bombed out of their minds. History courses and textbooks were rewritten to downplay the importance of Washington, Jefferson, Adams, and Madison and elevate progressive heroes like Malcolm X. More pages were consumed by a discussion of the Ku Klux Klan than the American Constitution. The Constitution and the Declaration of Independence were spurned as the scribblings of rich, white, male slaveowners. All white European males – from Columbus to Shakespeare—soon became targets of the professorial elite. Private property was condemned and all cultures – even those with abhorrent practices like human sacrifice – were judged of equal or even superior worth to our own.

Students graduating from public middle and high schools who already had received a flimsy and incomplete education about the history of the American Republic and the values that guided the Framers were now thrown into university classes unprepared for radical left indoctrination and unvaccinated against the crazy nostrums of their instructors. Had these children even heard of Montesquieu, the philosophical father of the concept of separation of powers? Had they been taught about John Locke, Edmund Burke, or John Randolph? Did they know about the Articles of Confederation, the Federalist Papers, or the genesis of the Bill of Rights? Had they studied anything about ancient Rome or ancient Greece and the impact these great civilizations had on our own Founding Fathers and their philosophy of government?

If you don't know who you are and where you came from, you can't be expected to fight to preserve your heritage. You are defenseless to the assaults of the nihilists. And that is where we are today. Statues and monuments being toppled, holidays abolished (remember when we had separate holidays for George Washington and Abraham Lincoln to commemorate their distinct contributions to our country?), streets and military bases renamed, and soon our cities that carry the names of the Catholic saints and were brought to the Americas by Christian missionaries will be renamed. Goodbye San Diego, San Francisco, and San Jose!

What is happening is a tragedy of incalculable proportions. It foretells a frightening future for all Americans. Can it be stopped or is it already too late? Can we retake our civilization and culture from those who have hijacked it? We will have a better idea come November 4.

MEDIA:

IT'S TIME TO BREAK UP BIG MEDIA

October 2, 2020

T HE CLEVELAND PRESIDENTIAL DEBATE WAS A DIS-
graceful spectacle unworthy of a great nation. However, it
was not disgraceful due to the behavior of the candidates (although
senile Joe Biden's insults were appallingly disrespectful to the
presidency). It was disgraceful due to the performance of the
so-called Commission on Presidential Debates and the moderator, Democrat Chris Wallace.

In reality, what occurred in Cleveland and what has occurred
in prior years under the control of the Commission was not a
debate. It was a joint press conference. A true debate would not
have the moderator consistently interrupting one of the candidates,
but not the other. A true debate would not permit the moderator
to cut off one of the candidates, but not the other. A true debate
would not permit the moderator to limit the discussion of relevant
issues. A true debate would not permit a moderator of obvious
political bias.

The chaos in Cleveland was simply the latest manifestation
of the deep-rooted and undeniable lack of even basic objectivity
on the part of the American news media. While the media, dominated by graduates of elite journalism schools like Columbia,

where liberal propaganda flourishes, has had a left bias as long as anyone can remember, it has become pathological in the era of Donald Trump. Entire volumes could be written on the media's systematic program of character assassination of the President and his administration over the last four years. There is no need to revisit that here. It has been so obvious it doesn't require a review.

What needs to be addressed is what to do about it.

Back in the early 1970s, then-Vice President Spiro Agnew became the first national public figure to take on the national press in a bare-knuckled manner. He was reacting to the media's shilling for American retreat in Vietnam and solidarity with draft card-burners and rioters burning down America's cities.

Agnew accurately described the three major networks (at that time) as being little more than a cabal of privileged elites who collaborated to create their own version of the news, which was then spoon-fed to the American public every evening at 7 pm. Agnew pointed out how the headlines and storylines were always in sync, never varying, but indicative of the fact that the so-called competitors CBS, ABC, and NBC actually conspired to feed the same narrative to the American people night after night.

Of course, what we face today is a far more serious concentration of power in the hands of a small corporate elite that dominates America's information system.

Today, 90 percent of U.S. media is controlled by just six media conglomerates: GE/Comcast (NBC, Universal), News Corp (Fox News, *Wall Street Journal, New York Post*), Disney (ABC, ESPN, Pixar), Viacom (MTV, BET, Paramount Pictures), Time Warner (CNN, HBO, Warner Bros.) and CBS (Showtime, NFL.com). The wealthiest man on the planet, Amazon's Jeff Bezos, owns the *Washington Post*. Two hundred thirty-two media executives control what media 330 million Americans consume. That's one media executive for every 1.4 million American consumers!

This media consolidation is compounded by the Big Tech monopoly in which the digital despots maintain Orwellian-like control of the Internet. Through Google, Yahoo, Facebook, YouTube, and Twitter, online news is controlled by just a handful of corporations whose accumulated wealth is greater than the Gross Domestic Product of most nations on Earth. The Big Tech monopolies determine what you can see and read on the Internet, manipulate algorithms to downgrade conservative news outlets on search engines, and outright censor content, determining what they believe is factual content. And most of these corporations lavishly fund the Democrat Party and its candidates, creating a yawning conflict-of-interest when it comes to their coverage of campaigns and elections.

The global corporations who control the news media and the Internet detest Donald Trump precisely because he is an anti-globalist. The global corporations seek to amass massive power and wealth by offshoring American jobs and onshoring cheap illegal immigrant labor. As Trump's policies are diametrically opposed to their agenda, they seek his destruction. The so-called reporters and journalists who vilify him and members of his administration are not reporters or journalists at all. They are simply paid PR hacks, doing the bidding of their corporate masters. They have no journalistic skills or ethics. Their goal is not to inform but to propagandize. They are no better than the Nazi Party hacks who served Joseph Goebbels in 1930s Germany.

At the turn of the 20th Century, railroad and oil monopolies led by corporate barons like John D. Rockefeller ruled the land, manipulating prices and driving farmers and small merchants out of business. A President named Theodore Roosevelt took them on. He took on the trusts and enacted anti-monopoly laws to curb their pernicious influence. The Supreme Court ruled that the Standard

Oil monopoly was a threat to the republic and must be immediately dissolved.

The situation is little different today, only the players have changed. It's not the oil companies or railroads or even the airlines or automobile manufacturers who are threats to the republic. The greatest threat to any nation is any group that controls and manipulates the free flow of news and information to rig elections and influence public policy. The debate in Cleveland was election interference on the part of NewsCorp employee Chris Wallace to bail out a doddering Democrat named Joe Biden. It was far greater than anything Russia ever did. The enemy is indeed within, not without.

What needs to happen now, in a Trump second term, is for Attorney General Bill Barr to dust off the antitrust laws and empower the antitrust division of the Justice Department to break up the Big Media and Big Tech monopolies as a threat to the republic. They must be declared monopolies in restraint of trade and once broken up, must be prohibited from re-organizing under other names. Their tax breaks and privileges should be revoked. And the libel and slander laws should be reformed to prevent these corporate flacks masquerading as journalists from hiding behind the First Amendment to shield them from the consequences of their lies.

Big Media and Big Tech want to take America down. It's time for America to take them down.

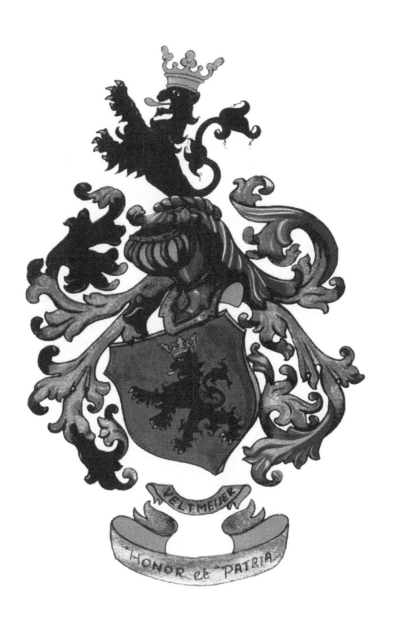

HOMELESSNESS:

OVERCOMING THE TRAGEDY OF HOMELESSNESS

September 10, 2019

U NLIKE MANY POLITICIANS WHO PONTIFICATE ON THE subject, I actually experienced homelessness as a young boy, living in the streets of South America. I was lucky. I was able to come to the United States and start a new life. I was fortunate my mother had a sister living in El Cajon who agreed to take me in.

When we examine the homeless crisis today, my experience can be instructive. I had a relative who enabled me to overcome my homeless state, go to school, work, and become successful. And this was in *another* country.

To what extent are our self-appointed homeless experts today (who seem to be experts in wasting taxpayer money on "solutions" that don't work) actually talking to the people living in the streets, trying to determine what landed them there and why? Everyone is different and every homeless person certainly has a different story to tell.

For example, how much effort is made to connect the homeless with family members and relatives, some of whom might be unaware of their situation and willing to help? The same could be said of previous employers, teachers, pastors, or even physicians.

How much time is spent actually learning the background of these unfortunates as any good social worker would do?

How about our churches, the historic houses of Christian charity, which were the main sources of assistance to those down on their luck until Big Government shoved them aside and decided to replace God with the Department of Health and Human Services?

Is simply building more housing the answer? Probably not. While the lack of affordable housing may be a factor, it isn't the main cause of homelessness. If it were, major cities in the Midwest and Rust Belt where housing is dirt-cheap would have no homeless problems at all. That's certainly not the case.

Of course, California's housing costs are astronomical. However, will replacing a $1 million home with an "affordable" home of half that amount really help the homeless eating out of garbage cans and sleeping on park benches? Of course not. Before one homeless person can even think about an "affordable" or "low income" house or apartment, he or she needs a job, needs to receive the proper medical or mental health care, drug rehabilitation, and needs the education and training required to offer an employer the skills the job requires.

Medical care. Mental health care. Drug rehab. Education and jobs. Those are the keys to overcoming homelessness. Sadly, it is true that most of the people living on our nation's streets suffer from mental illness or a drug problem. Changes in the way we have treated these conditions over the decades has resulted in releasing individuals into the general community rather than caring for them in group homes and other facilities where they can get "cleaned up" and ready for the real world again.

Sending a drug addict out into the streets after a month or two of rehab may only result in the cycle starting all over again. Many of our homeless are actually veterans, the finest our nation has to offer. It is a disgrace to see them living this way. Instead of spending billions on showering benefits on those who broke into our country illegally, let's redirect those funds to our homeless veterans, to help them find schooling and jobs or overcome any addictions they have fallen victim to. The same general principle applies to all of America's homeless.

As a legal immigrant myself, I can safely express my politically incorrect outrage that illegal immigrants are treated better than our fellow citizens who have lost jobs to cheap labor or bad trade agreements or been priced out of a decent education or become hooked on licit or illicit drugs, perhaps only out of the deep depression they suffer for what has happened to them. As a nation, as a state, as a city, let's resolve to be our brother's keeper. Let's start implementing policies that actually get the homeless off the streets and back to their families or churches or into classrooms and jobs, instead of dead-end handouts or "pie-in-the-sky" political promises that prevent them from helping themselves achieve a better life as I did.

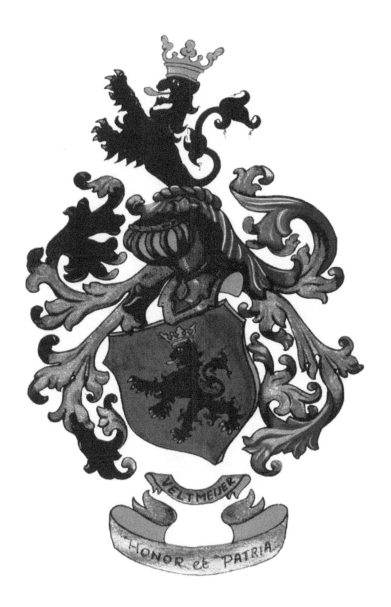

VELTMEIJER

HONOR et PATRIA

FEDERAL
RESERVE SYSTEM:

IS TRUMP RIGHT TO GO AFTER THE FED?

October 4, 2019

P RESIDENT TRUMP'S RECENT ATTACKS ON THE Federal Reserve and its interest rate policies have drawn more public attention to the actions of the nation's shadowy central bank than at any time since the great crash of 2008 or Ron Paul's campaigns for President a decade ago.

The President is correct in questioning the Fed's current approach to the economy. Raising interest rates too quickly following a long era of easy money can indeed cause the type of shock that can push a nation into recession. That's exactly what happened in 2007-08. Then-Fed chairman Alan Greenspan had pursued a low interest rate policy after 9/11, only to tighten rapidly after 2005, quintupling the federal funds rate from 1 percent to 5.25 percent in just four years. This contributed mightily to the subsequent mortgage crisis and housing collapse.

We saw such counterproductive actions just decades before. Paul Volcker's interest rate policies in the late 1970s and early 1980s raised rates to 21 percent, throwing the U.S. into the worst recession since the Great Depression and greatly complicating Ronald Reagan's plans to revive the economy. While Volcker did succeed in breaking the back of inflation, he almost destroyed the U.S. economy in the process.

The question the President should be asking is: Why is one individual (the Chairman of the Fed) granted so much power over the nation's economy? Why is a central bank that is unelected and has never been subjected to an independent audit permitted to exercise such control over the nation's money supply? This is a question that goes back to the early days of the American Republic.

One of the earliest battles over a central bank was waged between Thomas Jefferson and Alexander Hamilton. Small-government Jeffersonians denounced the idea of surrendering control of the nation's money to a privately owned banking monopoly. After all, does not the Constitution confer the power to "coin money and regulate the value thereof" to the people's elected representatives in the Congress? Nowhere in the Constitution is there mention of a central bank. However, the wealthy ruling elites have always desired a central bank because such a bank gave them a *carte blanche* to print money at will and lend money to debt-ridden governments *at interest*. That's why the Bank of England was established in 1694 and why Lord Rothschild was quoted as saying: "Give me control of a nation's money and I care not who makes the laws."

The Hamiltonians won the early skirmish and George Washington reluctantly agreed to charter the First Bank of the United States in 1791. It was authorized for twenty years. Anti-central bank President James Madison – Father of the Constitution – refused to renew it and let it die a well-deserved death. It was resurrected just five years later as the Second Bank of the United States, but became so thoroughly corrupted by crony capitalism that Andrew Jackson killed it off permanently in 1832.

The United States remained generally free of the central bank "vipers" (Jackson's appellation) until the creation of the Fed in

308

1913. Abraham Lincoln refused the bankers' loansharking terms during the Civil War and financed the war with interest-free United States Notes. After several artificially created economic "panics" in the post-Civil War era, the Rockefellers, Rothschilds, Morgans, and Warburgs devised a scheme to create a new central bank they would control, but camouflaged it in such a way as to imply it was a federal agency. The Federal Reserve most assuredly is not a part of the federal government. It is about as federal as Federal Express. While the President may appoint its Board of Governors, the regional Federal Reserve banks are privately owned.

Since the Fed was created, the dollar has lost about 97 percent of its value. The National Debt has skyrocketed from $3 billion to $22 trillion. Interest payments on the debt alone are more than the entire Federal Budget when Jimmy Carter was in the White House. Our economy has been locked in a "boom-bust" cycle involving either inflation or deflation, prosperity or recession – all as a result of money being created out of thin air to fund welfare and wars and the price-fixing of interest rate manipulation. The Fed presided over (and some argue, caused) the Great Depression followed by a series of smaller recessions, the hyperinflation of the 1970s, the dot.com bust of 2000, and the Crash of 2008. A great record for an institution set up to stabilize the nation's financial system! It's probably safe to say that the first ten individuals in the Cincinnati telephone directory could have done a better job managing the nation's economy than the so-called financial "geniuses" at the Fed.

Of course, what business does any individual or institution have in managing a free market economy? A free market economy is managed by millions of producers and consumers who interact on a daily basis, not the President, the Treasury Secretary, faceless bureaucrats, or central bankers.

If President Trump wants to get to the bottom of the money-printing and money-lending scam that is the Federal Reserve System, he should work for passage of Sen. Rand Paul's legislation to audit the Fed. It's time to rip the mask off America's most secretive, unaccountable, and unconstitutional body, a racket developed and designed to benefit the wealthy elites and ruling class while impoverishing the middle and working classes by destroying the value of their hard-earned dollars. He should then act decisively to begin the process of repealing the Federal Reserve Act of 1913, restoring full convertibility of the dollar to gold, and transferring authority to "coin money and regulate the value thereof" back to the people.

DEEP STATE:

IS IT TIME TO ABOLISH THE CIA?

October 8, 2019

E XACTLY ONE MONTH AFTER THE ASSASSINATION OF President John F. Kennedy, former President Harry Truman made an interesting observation about the Central Intelligence Agency which was published in the *Washington Post*. Truman wrote: "For some time I have been disturbed by the way the CIA has been diverted from its original assignment...It has become an operational and at times a policy- making arm of the Government. This has led to trouble and may have compounded our difficulties in several explosive areas."

Of course, the CIA was established under Truman in 1947, tasked with gathering, processing, and analyzing national security information from around the world. That limited role of intelligence gathering quickly morphed into the CIA taking on the role of a secret army, intervening throughout the world to overthrow governments, wage clandestine wars, and install compliant rulers.

As early as the Korean War, the CIA was sending agents into the North to recruit North Korean expatriates for guerrilla operations. In 1953, the CIA engineered a coup in Iran to oust the democratically elected government of Mohammed Mossadegh who was threatening British oil interests in that country. The CIA installed the Shah in Mossadegh's place, leading to twenty-five years of repression that led to the anti-American Islamic Revolution of 1979 and accounts for much of the enmity the Iranians hold toward the United States to this day. A year later, the spy agency was at it again, overthrowing the Arbenz government of Guatemala, which was threatening the massive land holdings of the United Fruit Company. Subsequent CIA meddling followed in Indonesia, the Democratic Republic of the Congo, and the Dominican Republic. In Indonesia, the CIA even used its own B-26 planes to bomb and strafe the nation in an attempt to oust leftist President Sukarno!

Of course, the CIA's 1961 attempt to overthrow Fidel Castro probably ranks as the most notorious of the agency's regime-changing activities. A rebel army was recruited and trained by the CIA – authorized by the Eisenhower and Kennedy Administrations – to take Castro out. However, at the last minute, Kennedy had a change of heart and denied the rebels the air support they needed to succeed. The resulting slaughter of the anti-Castro Cubans on the beaches of the Bay of Pigs was almost predictable. The CIA blamed Kennedy for the failure of the operation and Kennedy condemned the CIA, vowing to destroy the agency and scatter it to the winds.

John F. Kennedy was killed in Dallas on November 22, 1963. Most serious students of the assassination discount the Warren Commission whitewash and have offered convincing evidence that the CIA – or elements within that agency (possibly working with members of organized crime) — was responsible for Kennedy's death. The CIA's multifaceted adventures expanded greatly during the turbulent 1960s, from involvement in the brutal slayings of anti-Communist South Vietnamese President Diem and his brother in November 1963 to a variety of covert actions supporting the U.S. military throughout the Vietnam War, including a controversial plan to destroy the Vietcong infrastructure known as the Phoenix Program, as well as alleged drug-running out of the Burma Triangle. The CIA also was active on the home front, infiltrating antiwar and student organizations and conducting domestic surveillance.

Outrage over the CIA's extra-constitutional escapades reached a fever pitch in the mid-1970s, in the aftermath of Vietnam and the Watergate scandal as well as the 1973 overthrow of President Salvador Allende of Chile. The U.S. Senate established a special select committee headed by Sen. Frank Church of Idaho to investigate the agency's nefarious work. The committee revealed that far from being an intelligence-gathering service, the Central Intelligence Agency was actually engaging in foreign assassinations and regime change on a massive scale. It was also systematically violating the privacy rights of thousands of American citizens by intercepting mail, wiretapping, etc.

Despite the concerns raised by the Church Committee, the CIA continued on its merry way throughout the 1980s and beyond, from funneling $40 billion in weapons to the Afghan resistance to training the Nicaraguan Contras and mining that nation's ports.

Yet, in carrying out its actual designated mission of collecting intelligence around the world to enhance U.S. national security, the CIA has often dropped the ball. From failing to recognize the percolating Islamic Revolution in Iran in 1979 to its failures prior to 9/11 and its false claim that it was a "slam dunk" that Saddam Hussein had weapons of mass destruction, this agency has proved itself incompetent in its original assignment.

Now, over the last three years, we have seen the CIA – the very symbol of the so-called "Deep State" — engaged in a slow-motion coup to overthrow the President of the United States. The involvement of this agency and other intelligence and law enforcement agencies in fabricating the Russian collusion hoax based on phony dossiers from foreign agents is stuff of James Bond.

President Obama's CIA Director John Brennan – who voted for the Communist Party candidate for President in 1976 — has been possessed by a burning hatred of President Trump since before his election. The same goes for Obama's Director of National Intelligence James Clapper. These two individuals, along with disgraced FBI Director Jim Comey, constitute the triumvirate of treason that colluded with foreign governments and foreign intelligence services along with the Hillary Clinton campaign to infiltrate and spy on the Trump campaign and destroy the Trump presidency from the outset. Now, we learn that the so-called "whistleblower" who lacked any first-hand knowledge of the President's conversation with Ukraine's leader is a CIA officer! What a surprise!

The time has come for Congress to reassert its constitutional responsibility over the U.S. intelligence apparatus. These agencies have been discredited in the eyes of the American people and the world. They have little or no credibility left. Perhaps it is time to abolish the CIA and start over again. The American people do not want rogue spooks running secret wars with secret bank accounts and their own bomber squadrons. They don't want their tax money used for surreptitious plots to assassinate world leaders and topple foreign governments. The Constitution gives the power to declare war strictly to Congress, not the President, not the Secretary of State, and certainly not to the Central Intelligence Agency.

Let's hope when the final page is written in the saga of the Trump Russian collusion hoax, it will lead to a consensus that the CIA and its sibling agencies either return to their original intelligence functions or be dissolved entirely.

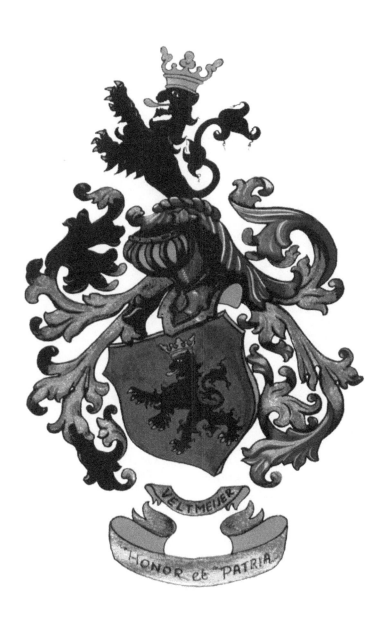

CLIMATE CHANGE:

CLIMATE CHANGE AND BACKDOOR SOCIALISM

December 30, 2019

SOCIALIST CONGRESSWOMAN ALEXANDRIA Ocasio-Big Mouth says the world will end in twelve years unless American taxpayers fork over $93 trillion to implement a "Green New Deal." At a cost of almost five times the size of the entire U.S. economy, this revolutionary program would transform the U.S. economy into a centrally planned command economy ruled by federal bureaucrats. Under AOC's scheme, the oil and gas industry would be deep-sixed, every building in America razed to the ground and rebuilt, meat consumption banned, and air travel abolished.

Obviously, only by handing over totally unprecedented and unconstitutional powers to the federal government could such a monstrosity be imposed upon the American people. Needless to say, millions of jobs would be eliminated, basic rights terminated, and an inflation of unparalleled intensity unleashed to pay for it. The "Green New Deal" would require the fundamental transformation of a basically free market American economy into a socialist economy where government, not millions of producers and consumers, make the decisions. It is frightening and it is absurd.

However, it is supposedly the answer to "climate change," that mind-numbing and life-altering threat to our very existence which is just around the corner. Of course, to the doomsayers, it has been around the corner for years now, but we seem to keep plodding along.

History is replete with the prophets of doom who have predicted imminent disaster if we didn't hand over power and money to them. Government's greatest control over people has always been to convince them that there's an existential crisis that demands their immediate and enlightened intervention. Such intervention usually ends in disaster, with the cure being far worse than the disease.

In the late 1960s, a Stanford professor named Paul Ehrlich wrote a widely discredited book called the *Population Bomb*, which predicted widespread famine throughout the world in the 1970s and 1980s due to overpopulation. He wrote: "In the 1970s, hundreds of millions of people will starve to death..." Never happened.

On the first Earth Day in 1970, Ehrlich warned that "in ten years all important animal life in the sea will be extinct. Large areas of coastline will have to be evacuated because of the stench of dead fish." In a 1971 speech, his crystal ball prophesied that "By the year 2000 the United Kingdom will be simply a small group of impoverished islands, inhabited by some 70 million hungry people." So much for Paul Ehrlich's talents as a clairvoyant. Jonathan Last called the *Population Bomb* "one of the most spectacularly foolish books ever published."

Ehrlich's solution for the non-crises he predicted: government control over population, including abortion and sterilization.

Ehrlich's "doom and gloom" view wasn't new. It hearkens back to the laughable theories of British economist Thomas Malthus in the 18th century, who also projected mass starvation caused by population growth outstripping food production. What Malthus didn't take into account was the incredible productivity of the free market system and modern agriculture technologies, which consistently produced food surpluses, not shortages.

In the late 1970s, a new Ice Age was all the rage. *Time* magazine ran a cover headline story in 1977 entitled "How to Survive the Coming Ice Age." Needless to say, again, no such phenomenon ever happened.

Today's hysteria over "climate change" appears to be little more than warmed-over Malthusianism with a big dose of power-seeking by advocates of total government.

In his outstanding new book, *The Case Against Socialism,* Kentucky Senator Rand Paul makes a number of important observations about global warming.

First of all, scientific opinion is far from unanimous, although the Left would have us believe it is. So-called "climate deniers" include science Nobel Laureates as well as a recipient of NASA's Medal for Exceptional Scientific Achievement. Only 36 percent of geoscientists and engineers believe that humans are creating a global warming crisis, according to a survey reported in the peer-reviewed *Organization Studies.* By contrast, a strong majority of the 1,077 respondents believe that nature is the primary cause of recent global warming and/or that future global warming will not be a very serious problem.

Apocalyptic predictions of polar bears disappearing and loss of the world's glaciers have proven to be false. NASA now reports that CO_2 emissions are actually "greening" the Earth, leading to higher yields in agriculture and forestry, and more efficient use of water by vegetation generally.

Senator Paul cites the so-called Milankovic cycles developed by a Serbian geophysicist and astronomer in the 1920s, which have never been disputed or disproved. Professor Milankovic claimed that changes in climate are actually related to changes in the earth's orbit and tilt.

Do the global warming fanatics have a hidden agenda? Is it really socialism with climate change just a façade?

In his book, Rand Paul references one Eric Holthaus, a columnist for *Grist,* who says dismantling capitalism is the "key requirement to maintaining civilization and a habitable planet." He also cites socialist Matthew Huber who writes in his essay, "Five Principles of a Socialist Climate Politics," that "the climate struggle is less about knowledge and more about a material struggle for power."

"Struggle for power." Let those words sink in. Is that the real agenda behind the climate change hysteria? We have to ask ourselves why so many self-avowed socialists have embraced what is little more than a questionable theory and why they have rolled out grandiose schemes to completely revolutionize the American economy into a socialist planned economy to address their concerns. Is it really necessary to destroy capitalism to reduce CO_2 emissions? Why are they not concerned about the chief polluters on the planet, Communist China and India?

While there are certainly well-intentioned people on both sides of this debate, we must never permit the AOCs and Bernie Sanders of the world to use this issue to impose backdoor socialism on an American nation that would reject socialism if offered in its pure, unvarnished form.

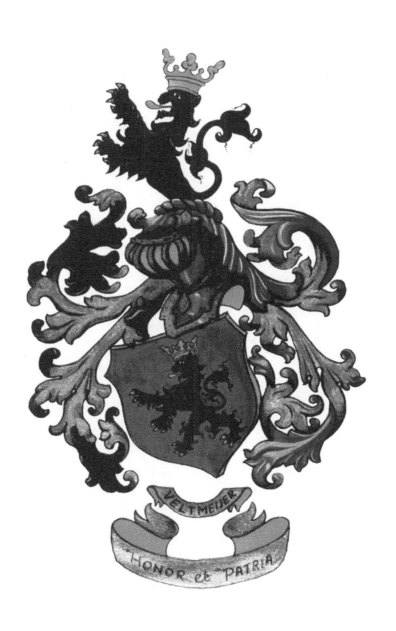

SOCIAL SECURITY:

QUO VADIS, SOCIAL SECURITY?

February 19, 2020

C LOCKING IN AT MORE THAN $1 TRILLION ANNUALLY, Social Security is the largest federal program in existence, consuming more than one-fifth of all federal dollars and representing 5 percent of Gross Domestic Product. It is also probably the most grandiose federal program ever enacted and has long been considered virtually sacrosanct, the so-called "third rail" of American politics.

Enacted in 1935 as the "crown jewel" of Franklin D. Roosevelt's New Deal Revolution, Social Security built on previous attempts to provide old-age pensions such as the programs of the Iron Chancellor Bismarck in 1880s Germany. During the Great Depression, the idea of providing supplemental income to senior citizens gained traction with the Townsend Plan, an idea advanced by an American physician, Dr. Francis Townsend, as a means of stimulating the U.S. economy. The Townsend Plan proposed giving every retired American over sixty $200 per month, which needed to be spent within thirty days. It would be funded by a 2 percent national sales tax.

FDR's plan was heavily influenced by Townsend but was financed with a payroll tax instead of a sales tax. With the program not kicking in until the age of sixty-five and life expectancy at that time less than age sixty-five, Social Security seemed a no-brainer. With forty-two people paying into the system for every one retiree, massive surpluses built up in the system, the so-called "Trust Fund." The payroll tax started at just 2 percent and was never to rise higher than 6 percent. Most people did not live long enough to collect benefits and if they did, their life span was shorter.

Designed as a "pay as you go" system, Social Security was demographically challenged from the beginning. Instead of individuals' "contributions" being invested in stocks, mutual funds, real estate or other economic assets promising a generous rate of return, the taxes paid the benefits of current recipients, making it more of a welfare or redistribution scheme than a retirement plan. It could only remain successful as long as a growing number of workers contributed at higher and higher tax rates to support a growing number of retired seniors living longer and longer lives. The so-called "surpluses" that developed in the early years due to a massive influx of "contributions" and limited payout dwindled as the politicians repeatedly raided the surpluses to fund other government programs, like endless wars abroad.

The politicians always saw Social Security as a way to win votes from the elderly and signed off on expanding the program in subsequent years, such as adding disability benefits under President Eisenhower in 1956, medical coverage through Medicare under LBJ in 1965, cost-of-living adjustments under Richard Nixon just before the 1972 election, and prescription drug coverage by President Bush in 2005. Payroll taxes kept rising to keep up with the growth of the program, the increased number of retirees and the declining numbers of workers to support the program. Today, the payroll tax is 15.3 percent (including Medicare) and the number of working Americans supporting it down to just 3.4 to every one retiree. With Americans having fewer children and the "baby boomers" living longer than ever, any program based on a "pay as you go" foundation is doomed to inevitable collapse. The program is currently "borrowing" from its fictitious $2.9 trillion "surplus" to pay current benefits (which essentially means swapping IOUs), but that will run out by 2035. At that point, taxes alone will cover only about 79 percent of benefits. That's when it will all hit the fan.

The tragedy of Social Security is that a well-intentioned plan to provide the elderly with additional retirement security in their golden years devolved— thanks to the vote-buying and manip-ulation of politicians – into a demographically and financially insolvent Ponzi scheme that can only pay benefits if new people enter the system and pay taxes. The program has served also to discourage four generations of Americans from taking personal responsibility for their retirement and saving accordingly, making the great majority of seniors almost totally dependent on their Social Security check for survival.

Back in 1964, Senator Barry Goldwater of Arizona – the lib-erty-loving Republican candidate for President – was one of the very few political leaders at the time to sound the alarm bell about Social Security. Contrary to the phony propaganda thrown against him by LBJ and the national media, Goldwater never advocated abolishing Social Security. He simply suggested that Americans should be left free to invest privately for their own retirement if they saw fit. He objected to the mandatory nature of the program, not the program itself. He believed that if working Americans could find a better alternative to Social Security, through a mutual fund, annuity, or some other retirement plan, they should be freed of the burden of the payroll tax.

In recent years, many more politicians have come to agree with Goldwater. Even President George W. Bush advocated allowing Americans to re-assign a portion of their payroll tax to a private retirement plan. The Democrats, however, ever eager to pander for votes, ensured that such a sensible idea never saw the light of day. Instead, they are content to just support raising payroll taxes higher and higher to fund a broken system, regressive taxes that hurt low-income wage-earners hardest.

Of course, the enormous popularity of IRAs and 401k retirement plans in recent decades points to the inherent superiority of private sector solutions over those of the public sector. Individuals invested in stock-based IRAs can see an average annual return of more than 7 percent as opposed to 2 percent or less in the government bonds invested in by the Social Security "trust fund." That's why so many Americans have chosen to participate in these plans, while still having to pay a high payroll tax for benefits many of them doubt they will ever receive. It's high time Americans are freed from the albatross of the Social Security payroll tax and allowed to invest those funds in private retirement accounts. This is what Chile did back in the 1980s when they reformed their Social Security program. In exchange, younger Americans so invested will relinquish their rights to Social Security benefits when they retire and should be repaid whatever they have already paid in. The only exception should be those Americans fifty and older. They should be guaranteed whatever benefits they are owed. By permitting (but not requiring) younger workers to invest privately for their old age, a new economic boom would be realized, with hundreds of billions of dollars becoming available for new investments throughout the country.

Social Security may be the biggest and boldest federal program ever devised with an enormous voting constituency behind it. Yet, we must put the politics aside to avoid financial calamity and ensure retirement security for all Americans in the coming years.

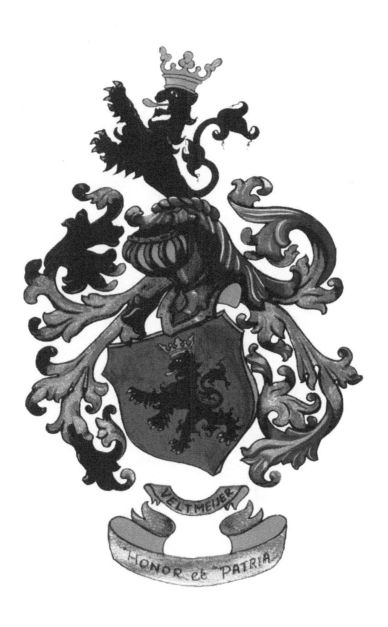

LAW ENFORCEMENT:

THE HIDDEN AGENDA BEHIND "DEFUND THE POLICE"

August 3, 2020

B ACK IN THE 1960s, THERE WAS A CAMPAIGN launched by conservative political activists called "Support Your Local Police....and Keep Them Independent." During that turbulent period in U.S. history, law enforcement was under heavy attack, just as today. In the midst of riots and civil unrest associated with the civil rights movement and the Vietnam War, police officers were victimized for attempting to maintain order by violent radical left-wing groups like the Black Panthers, the Weather Underground and others. Unfortunately, as is the case today, some police officers were stereotyped as racists because of the actions of some of their brethren in the then-segregationist South.

The "Support Your Local Police" campaign was sparked by a desire to not only offer public support for law enforcement at a time it was under attack, but to preserve the concept of local autonomy and the independence of local police from the control of an all-powerful central government in Washington, D.C. Throughout history, dictatorships have quickly acted to secure their power by confiscating firearms in private hands and abolishing local law enforcement and placing it under the control of the central government or the party. This is what happened in Nazi Germany, for example.

The fact is that as long as local police forces exist, there is some check on the ability of the central government to oppress the population. A city police department under the authority of the elected mayor and city council could refuse to enforce a federal order to confiscate privately owned firearms, for example. A county sheriff is the highest law enforcement authority in that jurisdiction and can refuse to enforce laws that he finds are illegitimate or unlawful. A number of California sheriffs, for example, have said they will decline to enforce Governor Newsom's unconstitutional "edicts" regarding the mandatory usage of face masks. Others have organized into movements vowing to defy gun control legislation. By taking an oath of allegiance to the Constitution, they are duty-bound to refuse to obey political orders that violate our nation's guiding principles.

The very existence of independent, locally controlled police and sheriff's agencies is a major stumbling block in the way of power-hungry politicians who would seek to consolidate total control over the population. What they seek is a federal police force instead. This would be the most dangerous development that could occur in any free nation.

In recent months since the George Floyd incident, the attacks on the police have again moved into overdrive, but let no one believe it is simply motivated by a desire to end police brutality. Ending an occasional abuse or purging a few bad officers from a given department is not a justification for "defunding" the police entirely or slashing their budgets by millions of dollars or all but handcuffing officers in the face of violence and terrorism. Imagine your home is being broken into at 2 am and you're expected to call a social worker instead of a cop to deal with the situation. Completely insane.

Of course, the true facts simply do not support the false narrative that this nation is being overrun by rogue cops abusing and brutalizing civilians, be they black, brown or white. The truth is that deaths of unarmed people at the hands of police are rare. According to the FBI and the *Washington Post*, 1,004 individuals were killed by law enforcement officers in the U.S. last year. As Santa Barbara County Sheriff Bill Brown observed: "The overwhelming majority of those deaths were justifiable homicides committed by officers defending their lives or the lives of other people." Of the 1,004 who were killed, forty-one (4 percent) were unarmed. Of those forty-one, nineteen were white and nine were black. The remaining thirteen were either Latino or "other," including Asians and Native Americans. Since 2015, the number of such police shootings has remained steady at around 1,000 annually, so there has hardly been a surge. Critics of the police are quick to point out that 23 percent of those shot and killed by police are African-Americans when they only make up 13 percent of the population. Yet, African-Americans make up 53 percent of known homicide offenders and commit about 60 percent of robberies. Would the Left suggest we now establish racial quotas for criminal conduct?

The goal of the Left is simply to dissolve local law enforcement and replace it with a militarized federal police force empowered to run roughshod over states, counties, cities, and towns. You will be stripped of your right to elect your county sheriff, or in some cities, your chief of police. By defunding and hamstringing officers, the Left will unleash more crime and mayhem in our streets, leading a desperate population to demand federal action to quell the turmoil. Enter Top Cop Nancy Pelosi or Adam Schiff, who will be only too willing to oblige. It is true that President Trump and the Justice Department have acted to send some federal law enforcement agents into cities like Portland, but that was as a last resort to protect federal property, not to supplant and replace local police. Of course, the radical Left mayors of Portland and other cities are doing everything in their power to shut down the police and encourage the rioting and looting as a way to blame the President and throw the election to senile Joe Biden.

If we as Americans permit our local cops to be ridiculed, mocked, persecuted, assaulted, and killed, we will be paving the way for a new heavy-handed form of federal police power run from Washington, D.C. It will be the end of local control and local sovereignty and will pave the way for dictatorship in America. So, to resurrect the slogan from the 1960s, "Let's Support our Local Police and Keep Them Independent."

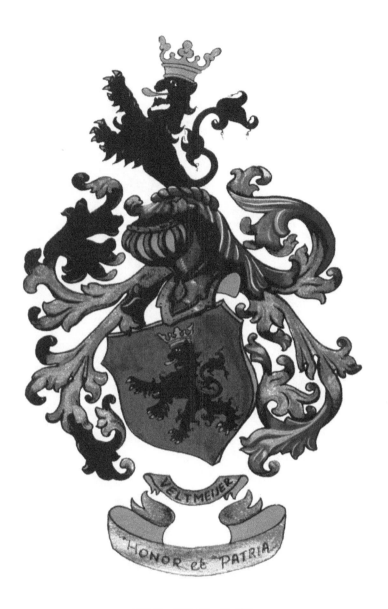

PUBLIC
EMPLOYEE UNIONS:

IT'S TIME TO REIN IN THE PUBLIC EMPLOYEE UNIONS

March 24, 2021

A RECENT REPORT IN *FORBES* AGAIN BRINGS THE American taxpayer's attention to another gigantic fiscal emergency-in-waiting: the unfunded liabilities of state and local governments due to the unfunded pension liabilities of the public employee unions. According to former California Assemblyman Chuck DeVore, these unfunded liabilities now exceed $5.2 trillion, more than the size of the entire federal budget. In California, this unfunded liability amounts to more than $86,000 per household. In Alaska, it's over $100,000. Nationwide, it's about $50,000 per household. Let's remember that's for the retirement of government employees; it doesn't build one school, one hospital, one airplane, or one ship.

The emergence of public employee unions is itself a relatively new phenomenon, starting in Wisconsin in 1959 and then spreading across the country to include teachers, clerks, firefighters, prison guards, and the police. In California, public employees got the "right" to bargain collectively during Jerry Brown's first administration in the mid-1970s. Today, California has an estimated $846 billion in unfunded pension liabilities.

We know that it is an inherent conflict-of-interest to allow politicians whose elections are funded by public sector unions to vote on the pay and benefit packages proposed by those unions. Yet, that is what is happening all across America and has been for decades. Have you ever heard of schemes such as 3 percent at thirty? That means a government employee, for example, can retire after thirty years (perhaps at age fifty-five or maybe younger) and earn – as his pension — 3 percent of the highest wage he was paid for each of those thirty years or 90 percent of his top salary working. Have you ever seen a deal like that in private industry? One state employee in Massachusetts took home $308,000 in his annual pension. Almost 80,000 retired government workers in California are collecting pensions of over $100,000 per year.

Due to the way that "defined benefit" pension programs are funded in the public sector, the retirements of public employees are heavily dependent on investment returns in the stock market. As Assemblyman DeVore states:

> *"In good times, pension fund investment income from Wall Street and other investment pours in, making the pension fund look fiscally sound. Politicians are reluctant to salt away added funds when the pension balance sheet looks strong. But in bad times, when investment returns go negative, government income also tends to be weak, leaving legislators with little appetite to put more money in to the pension fund."*

When the stock market collapses and local governments are financially strapped, who is on the hook for these obligations? It is you and me, the American taxpayer. Taxpayer support of state pensions for teachers rose from $611 million in 2001 to $3.5 billion in 2010 at the height of the Wall Street crash. In the city of San

Jose, pension expenses more than tripled between 2001 and 2010. This led to Mayor Chuck Reed's successful campaign to reform pensions two years later. What happens when local governments are forced to bail out these enormous retirement liabilities: less money for essential public services like libraries, roads, parks, and general maintenance or the inevitable tax increases.

It is estimated that these unions spend in excess of $1 billion annually at the federal, state, and local levels to keep the pensions rolling along. And these same unions will fight ferociously against any political leaders or initiatives who seek to upend their lucrative system. Just ask former Governor Arnold Schwarzenegger or the proponents of paycheck protection. The teachers' unions are especially notorious as they resist any attempts to improve public education and insist on an ossified adherence to the status quo. They have resisted tenure reform, increased teacher testing, better credentialing, and, of course, school choice. They claim to represent teachers, but really only represent their own highly compensated union bosses. Instead of championing our kids in the classroom, the NEA and AFT send about 95 percent of their union-confiscated dues to Democrats and engage in campaigns to repeal Proposition 13 in California. The California Teachers' Association donated almost $1.2 million to Gavin Newsom in his 2018 campaign for the state's top position.

State and local governments have been writing blank checks to the public sector unions for too long. Why do we accept legalized bribery in the form of their political contributions to the favored politicians who negotiate their contracts? As it's actually the taxpayers who are paying the bills, why aren't taxpayer advocates also at the negotiating table? At least when the UAW sits down with General Motors executives to hammer out their new contract, they are actually across the table from the folks who are signing their paychecks.

With this nation's debt on a glide path to $30 trillion in a few years, can we afford to be sacrificing our fiscal stability on an altar of unsustainable public pensions? Should our hard-working government employees continue to be victimized by a system that could eventually wind up leaving them high and dry, with no money to sustain them in their retirement years? And do the public employee unions have the right to continue in engage in reckless political lobbying and campaigning, despite the 2018 Supreme Court decision and even against the wishes of many of their own members? We need some answers to these questions and we need them now.

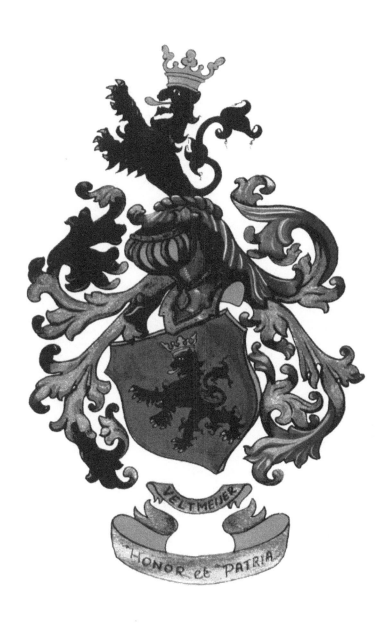

ELECTORAL REFORM:

MANDATING ELECTION INTEGRITY

February 25, 2021

A S A CONSEQUENCE OF THE QUESTIONABLE RESULTS of the November 3 presidential election, voter integrity laws and election reform should be the first order of business for the new Congress and the fifty state legislatures.

Few nations in the world conduct their elections in such a haphazard, schizophrenic manner as the United States. That explains why so many Americans doubt the results of last November's election.

It is unacceptable and unfathomable how the greatest nation in the history of the world cannot conduct its elections in a fair, transparent manner. Why were ballots still being counted in Congressional races three months after the election? Why did the battleground states all decide to stop counting ballots at the same time on election night? Why were observers thrown out of vote-counting centers in violation of the law? Why were state legis-latures unconstitutionally circumvented to make eleventh-hour changes to voting procedures?

These are questions that must be addressed and addressed soon before the public's faith in our democratic processes evaporate permanently.

The first issue that needs to be examined is the very day established in 1845 by the 28th Congress as the day on which we elect presidential electors. That day was assigned as "the Tuesday after the first Monday in November." Yet, what has occurred in recent years? Voters are increasingly being permitted in many states to vote weeks and even months before the date assigned by statute nearly 200 years ago. In the recent election, some states permitted voters to cast ballots as early as September! How is this not a clear and blatant violation of the law? And it is illogical as well. How can voters make a sound decision on the candidates weeks before the election, *before* they have received all the latest information they need to make a judicious choice?

Politics is chock-full of late-breaking developments – including the presidential debates and the Hunter Biden laptop scandal. Yet, voters are now allowed to vote before they have been exposed and given an opportunity to assimilate these late developments. In 1980, there was a huge swing to Ronald Reagan after the final presidential debate at the end of October. Could that have happened in 2020? We know now that a significant number of voters said they would not have voted for Joe Biden if they had known about the Hunter laptop fiasco. If we are to restore voter integrity, the first action that needs to be taken is to ensure that ballots are cast only on the designated day of voting.

The second issue is the matter of voter identification. Most nations of the world, including France, Israel, Mexico, Iceland, Germany, Norway, and Northern Ireland require some form of photo identification for a citizen to vote. This is only common sense. If only citizens are permitted to vote, how can we not demand that this citizenship is verified at the ballot box? We know that millions of individuals who are non-citizens (including both illegal immigrants and green card holders) have been illegally voting for years. This crisis has been worsened by the easy voter registration procedures now promoted in many states at their DMVs when individuals apply for driver's licenses. It is imperative that voter ID be mandated at the federal level for *every* state.

Third, the process for absentee or mail-in voting must be drastically reformed. Once upon a time, an individual could vote absentee only if he specifically requested an absentee ballot from his county registrar due to that individual having an excuse (i.e., being out-of-state on Election Day, etc.). In the 1990s, the laws were relaxed in California, for example, to allow almost anyone to apply for an absentee ballot, regardless of their status or condition. Then, California moved to something called "Permanent Vote-by-Mail" in which even the application was eliminated. And, in 2020, we discovered "COVID-voting" in which states just mailed a ballot to everyone on the voter rolls, even if those individuals were dead, had moved, or were otherwise ineligible to vote. Many people received multiple ballots, leading to widespread fraud. There are credible allegations of ballots being printed in different states or even countries and shipped around the nation last year where "boiler rooms" were utilized by the Democrats to fill in these fake ballots for Joe Biden. Of course, wide-open mail-in voting leads to this kind of massive abuse, as even former President Jimmy Carter observed. Mail-in voting needs to return to absentee voting, where a ballot is issued *only* upon receipt of a valid application and excuse. Ballot "harvesting," "drop-off" boxes and similar schemes must be prohibited by law. Even in a pandemic, if people can stand outside Costco, WalMart and Target, they can stand to wait to vote. It is just as important, arguably much more so.

Finally, the problems associated with electronic voting must be confronted. Most nations in the world (209 out of 227 to be exact) vote by paper ballot. That should be the case in the United States as well. Canada, for example, has long voted by paper ballot and counts its votes in a matter of a few hours and with great efficiency. In the United States, where ballots are cast by machine, counting goes on – in some cases – for days, weeks, and even months. It makes us the laughingstock of the planet. As far back as 1988, liberal media icon Dan Rather questioned whether "the fix" could be put on a national election through electronic voting machines and was told by the late Princeton University Professor Howard J. Strauss: "Get me a job with the company that writes the software for the program. Then I'd have access to one-third of the votes. Is that enough to fix a general election?" Strauss also stated: "When it comes to computerized elections, there are no safeguards. It's not a door without locks, it's a house without doors."

Of course, that was thirty years ago and technology is far more advanced today than it was then, meaning that computerized election fraud is probably more widespread and sophisticated today than back then. We can recall Democrats raising objections to the Diebold voting machines in Ohio during the 2004 presidential election, just as the Trump campaign exposed the machinations of Dominion in 2020. The fact is that electronic voting can be hacked, manipulated, connected to the Internet and otherwise made to switch votes and alter tabulations. The only safe course is to return to paper ballots cast and counted at the precinct level with observers present and watching. Voters should receive a paper receipt indicating how they voted so if there are any challenges, they can verify whether their vote was counted and registered as cast. Again, this needs to be *mandated* at the federal level.

America's election systems have been traditionally decentralized with the states primarily responsible for how those systems are run and elections conducted. However, due to the shenanigans encountered in the 2020 election, this decentralization needs to be reexamined. While it may be acceptable to have the states in control of their own local elections, we should and will require some kind of national standardization in federal elections to prevent a replay of what went down on November 3, 2020. And the state legislatures need to reclaim their constitutional authority (Article II, Section 1) to name presidential electors, so we don't have another spectacle of state legislators running to the Vice President at the last minute, asking to recertify their votes. These are actions unbecoming of the world's greatest republic.

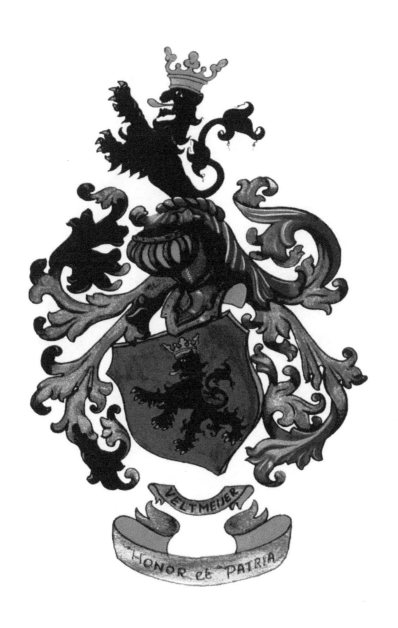

VELTMEUER

HONOR et PATRIA

THE BIDEN "PRESIDENCY":

JANUARY 20, 2021: THE FALL OF THE REPUBLIC

January 21, 2021

S ENILE JOE BIDEN WAS INSTALLED AS "PLACEHOLDER President" of the United States by more than 30,000 troops and a massive array of military hardware, yet hardly any regular American citizens attended as in past presidential inaugurations. Hastily placed flags replaced people in the name of COVID, but the swamp was present in force, including outgoing Vice President Mike Pence whose political career is over but who will undoubtedly receive a seven-figure job as a lobbyist for corporate interests in bed with Communist China. The January 20 event in Fortress D.C. was chillingly reminiscent of some Latin American or Middle Eastern despotism, not a constitutional republic.

Of course, Biden is simply a corrupt puppet playing a temporary role. He has no ideology other than loyalty to the almighty dollar. He will soon be moved out of office by Nancy Pelosi under the guise of the 25th Amendment to pave the way for Kamala Harris, who – based on her background and political associations – will arguably be America's first communist "president."

With control of the White House, the House of Representatives, and the Senate, the Radical Left is now fully empowered to launch the first of a series of Stalinist-like purges aimed at crushing all political opposition and constitutional liberties in America. This is their agenda and they are not concealing it.

Over the last several months, we have seen Big Tech engage in massive suppression of our First Amendment rights, including censoring the elected President of the United States who had over 80 million Twitter followers. Numerous other conservative leaders and journalists were shut down by Jack Dorsey and Mark Zuckerberg. Left-wing media personalities openly called for shutting down conservative media outlets, including Fox News. CNN demanded cable companies ban Fox as well as OANN and Newsmax. Giant corporations stopped all contributions to Republican officeholders and banned the sales of products by Trump-supporting business owners. Hitlerian calls for rounding up Trump supporters, establishing communistic neighborhood spying committees, and talk of new "domestic terrorism" legislation to disarm Trump supporters emerged. Officials at the Public Broadcasting System spoke openly of seizing the children of conservatives and placing them in "reeducation camps." Trump supporters have been fired from jobs or expelled from school. Lists are being compiled by the Left of people who innocently placed a Trump sign in their front yards. Social media accounts are being scoured for any comments reflecting support or sympathy for President Trump and his America First agenda. There are calls to purge Republicans from the military and law enforcement and to expel Republican members of Congress who supported the electoral vote challenge. Some have urged placing Senators Cruz and Hawley on "no-fly" lists as if they were terrorists.

This is how it starts.

This type of hyperventilated political rhetoric is typical in dictatorships just before the purges begin. You must demonize your political foes and make the general population fear their families, friends, and neighbors. Honest political debate or discussion is no longer permitted if it challenges the Left's dogma. Think of the Reign of Terror in France during the 1790s, Josef Stalin's purges in the 1930s, and Mao's Cultural Revolution during the 1960s.

It would appear that the current revolutionaries who compose the so-called Biden Administration and their allies in the propaganda mainstream media draw their inspiration most clearly from Mao, the greatest mass murderer in the history of the world, with nearly 70 million deaths attributed to his maniacal rule. While the 21st century "Red Guards" of AOC, Bernie Sanders, and Kamala Harris preach "democracy," they are actually its most deadly enemies. What this new communist regime in Washington, D.C., seeks is nothing less than the overthrow of America's constitutional republic and the abolition of the Bill of Rights. They detest any system bold enough to say our rights come from our Creator, rather than government. Their agenda is to replace our Bill of Rights with their own charter, which is patterned after Stalin's Soviet Constitution in which you only receive those rights bestowed upon you by the state and which can be just as easily taken away by the state.

In Communist China, the fanatical Red Guards rampaged through the cities and countryside, waving Mao's little red book, as they smashed statues, tore down historical statues and shrines, dragged intellectuals, poets, and writers out of their homes, and persecuted and killed anyone they suspected of harboring independent thoughts or ideas. Twenty million perished.

Terrifying days lie ahead for all Americans, especially for those who are believing Christians, gun owners, or any of the 75 million individuals who voted for Donald Trump. The Left smells blood and they are coming after you. They want you stripped of your rights, your guns, your education, or your businesses or jobs if you disagree with them. Ultimately, they would prefer you dead or in a concentration camp. Their shock troops – like Hitler's S.S. – are called Antifa and Black Lives Matter, and they will surely unleash new ones to terrorize and intimidate their opponents into silence and submission.

America is no longer at a tipping point. Tragically, it has tipped thanks to massive vote fraud in the November 2020 election. President Trump heroically held back the barbarians for four years. But now they are free to run loose and subject America to the final, fundamental transformation to a one-party totalitarian police state that Barack Obama promised a decade ago. We are now there. May God have mercy on the United States of America and deliver us from the untethered evil about to invade every state, town, and neighborhood across this land.

RESIST OR SUBMIT?

January 28, 2021

S ENILE JOE BIDEN'S VACUOUS "INAUGURAL ADDRESS" was filled with speechwriter- composed platitudes and empty words about "unity" which were carefully designed to hoodwink gullible Americans. For "unity" itself means nothing if it's a false unity based on errors or lies. It is equally without merit if – instead of meaning to seek cooperation, conciliation, and compromise – it simply means unifying to the left-wing agenda of Biden and his radical left-wing handlers. And, based on his Executive Orders and actions since January 20, it is obvious what Joe means by "unity": it means the 75 million Americans who voted for President Trump better submit or else. Nothing the Pretender President has done since that day indicates any desire or willingness to extend the olive branch to Republicans in Congress or supporters of President Trump.

The totalitarian Left – as inheritors of the bloody legacies of the French, Bolshevik and Maoist Revolutions – believes in "unity" about as much as the Communists believed in the "peace" they always preached about. For "peace" in the Marxist lexicon does not mean the absence of war, but the cessation of all oppo- sition to their rule. And, unity, in the Biden lexicon means the subjugation of all political dissent to the Left's platform. Do as we say and there will be unity. Defy us and we will come after you with everything in our arsenal.

How do patriots respond to the arrival of a totalitarian regime in Washington, D.C? Do we resist or do we submit and surrender our birthright as free men and women in the land purchased by the blood of our forebears? Submission is unquestionably not an option. Yet, what should full-scale resistance look like? Here are some ideas.

First of all, we must make ruthless and uninterrupted use of the courts to stifle, stymie, and stop the Biden regime's agenda for revolutionary change. This means Congress members, Governors, state legislators and others with standing to challenge every EO coming out of the Biden-occupied White House, from cancelling the Keystone XL pipeline to destroying girls' sports to throwing open the borders. We must raise the funds required to fight and win these courts cases, especially in front of the nearly 300 newly-minted Trump federal judges. We should wage unceasing war at the judicial level on every insane mandate or decree that comes from the "Red Diaper Babies" running the Biden show.

Second, we need to organize at the grassroots level to engage in massive peaceful civil disobedience to the Biden regime, taking a leaf from the Civil Rights efforts of the 1960s. From mask mandates to forced vaccinations to looney gender "fluidity" schemes, people simply should refuse *in masse* to cooperate in the surrender of our republic.

Third, boycotts. We should all begin undermining China Joe and his ChiCom-loving cronies and colleagues by refusing to purchase goods from Communist China, period. Drive a stake in the heart of the Chinese economy and military and Joe and Hunter's ill-gotten profits. If you can't find "Made in the USA" buy an item from India or South Korea which are at least democracies that don't murder their own people. These boycotts should extend to American corporations – such as Marriott, Kohl's, Wayfair, and Bed, Bath and Beyond, which are cutting off political contributions to Republican candidates or refusing to sell the products of businesses that support President Trump, like Mike Lindell's *My Pillow*. Just shop somewhere else, anywhere else. If you carry an Amazon credit card, tear it up and stop buying from Amazon period in response to pushing Parler off their server. Give that business to your local brick and mortar merchants who have been crushed so badly by the lockdowns. And, of course, get off Facebook and Twitter which are the regime's organs of political censorship. You lived without them before, you can live without them again. A decade ago, you never even heard of them. Send Jack Dorsey and Mark Zuckerberg back to their parents' garage.

Fourth, get out of the public schools. Stop letting your children be indoctrinated in anti-Americanism and the glories of socialism. Send them to a Christian or parochial school or, if you can't afford it, home school. The schools and universities have been the main sources of the Marxist infection contaminating our society. Grab your kids and flee.

Fifth, build our own infrastructure. It's long past time conservatives divorce themselves from the left-wing media culture. We need to build our own TV networks, news channels, cable systems, film production companies, newspapers, publishing houses, and social media channels. We also need to build our own financial platforms, banks, investment houses, and credit card companies. Sell off stock in companies that seek to destroy us and destroy America, invest in pro-American companies like *My Pillow*. We need to send a clear and unmistakable message to Big Business, Big Media, and Big Tech – silence us or curry favor with the Chinese Communist Party and we will disconnect you for good because we don't and won't need you anymore.

Finally, put the states back in charge of the union. Encourage state legislators to invoke "nullification" and "interposition" to defy unconstitutional federal rules and mandates coming down from Washington, D.C. Follow the example of some states and local communities declaring Second Amendment "sanctuaries." Establish state border patrols to enforce immigration law and deny federal authorities jurisdiction over the citizens of your states just like California and other "blue" states deny federal immigration officers jurisdiction over illegal immigrants in their states. Withhold tax monies from Washington. If the Biden regime continues down the path of a freedom-erasing totalitarianism, consider outright secession from the federal union, something not prohibited anywhere in the United States Constitution.

Two and a half centuries ago, the American colonists were in a not-so-dissimilar situation in regard to the British Empire. At the time, Patrick Henry declared: "Is life so dear, or peace so sweet, as to be purchased at the price of chains and slavery? Forbid it, Almighty God! I know not what course others may take; but as for me, give me liberty or give me death!" These immortal words can be justly applied to our current crisis. Will you resist or submit?

DR. JAMES VELTMEYER

Against ALL Odds

D R. JAMES VELTMEYER HAD AN ALMOST IMPOSSIBLE journey to his current status as one of the San Diego region's most well-respected doctors. Born in South America in 1968, his family became homeless when his father abandoned his mother. Dr. Veltmeyer's earliest recollections were living on the streets of Ecuador and going days without eating, sometimes being assigned the task of pleading for a few bread rolls at the local *panaderia* and often sacrificing his share, so there was enough for all his brothers and sisters to eat.

When Dr. Veltmeyer turned eleven, his mother made the heart-breaking decision to send him to live with an aunt in the United States. After a two-year effort, he obtained a visa and started his new life in San Diego County. At age nineteen, he became the sole provider for his family when his mother joined him to live in San Diego. Long motivated by his personal desire to help those in need, he then began chasing his dream of becoming a doctor by attending school full time and working multiple jobs to make ends meet.

Having such a challenging childhood might have discouraged others, but Dr. Veltmeyer was determined to make a difference, not just for himself but also for others.

After graduating from medical school, he completed his residency with UC San Francisco, becoming chief resident and overseeing thirty-five doctors. From there, he began his career at SGH Hospital in La Mesa and became Chair of the Department of Family Medicine.

As Chair, Dr. Veltmeyer oversaw over 200 physicians and was recognized as one of San Diego's leading physicians and surgeons. Known for going to extra lengths for his patients, he often faced cases written off by other physicians as hopeless and secured the extraordinary medical intervention that saved their lives. He took home numerous awards, including San Diego County's award for "Top Doctor" five years in a row, and in 2018 was named a "California Hero" by the California State Senate. He is also the host of the podcast program "Physician on a Mission," and his OpEds have appeared in publications across America, including *The Washington Times*.

Dr. Veltmeyer and his wife Laura are the proud parents of two children, Olivia and Landon. When not practicing medicine or spending time with his family, he is an avid sportsman. He enjoys surfing on San Diego's world-renowned beaches, skiing, playing golf, tennis and chess.

Dr. Veltmeyer is a shining example of the American Dream, overcoming huge obstacles to achieve success and reputation in his overall life and profession. He did this through religious faith, hard work, a commitment to build a better life for himself and his family, and a deep personal dedication to the founding principles of his adopted country, the United States of America. He believes faith and freedom can help even the most disadvantaged individuals reach for the stars and realize their hopes and dreams. Only in America.